LOW-CARB RECIPES COOKBOOK

A Proven Companion For Optimal Health And Weight Loss With Simple Dishes

Derek Klein

TABLE OF CONTENTS

Introduction **10**

Chapter One **14**

What Is a Low-Carb Diet? **14**

  Benefits Of A Low-Carb LifeStyle 17

  Understanding Net Carbs 19

Chapter Two **23**

Mouth-Watering Breakfast Recipes **23**

  1. Spinach And Feta Omelette 23

  2. Mushroom And Cheddar Scrambled Eggs 25

  3. Smoked Salmon And Cream Cheese Omelette 27

  4. Bacon And Spinach Scrambled Eggs 29

  5. Caprese Omelette 31

  6. Almond Flour Pancakes 32

  7. Coconut Flour Waffles 34

  8. Cream Cheese Pancakes 36

  9. Keto Cinnamon Roll Waffles 38

  10. Lemon Ricotta Pancakes 40

  11. Sugar-Free Maple Bacon 42

  12. Low-Carb Breakfast Sausage 43

  13. Low-Carb Ham Steak 45

  14. Low-Carb Canadian Bacon 46

  15. Low-Carb Steak And Eggs 47

Delicious Lunch Recipes **49**

  1. Grilled Chicken Breast With Avocado Salad 49

  2. Low-Carb Turkey Lettuce Wraps 51

  3. Tuna Salad With Celery Sticks 53

  4. Zucchini Boats With Turkey And Cheese 54

5. Cauliflower Fried Rice With Shrimp   56

6. Keto Cobb Salad   58

7. Chicken Caesar Salad with Romaine Lettuce 60

8. Low-Carb Chicken Quesadilla with Veggies 62

9. Baked Salmon With Green Beans And Almonds   64

10. Pork Chop With Roasted Veggies And Pesto   66

11. Low-Carb Chicken And Bacon Salad   68

12. Grilled Chicken Breast With Roasted Veggies   70

13. Spinach And Feta Stuffed Chicken Breast 72

14. Turkey And Cheese Roll-Ups With Lettuce 74

15. Chicken And Avocado Wrap With Lettuce And Tomato   76

Satisfying Dinner Recipes   78

1. Grilled Steak With Roasted Garlic Mashed Cauliflower   78

2. Baked Chicken Breast With Spinach, Feta, And Sun-Dried Tomatoes   80

3. Pork Tenderloin With Apple Cider Jus And Roasted Vegetables   82

4. Low-Carb Beef And Mushroom Gravy Over Cauliflower Mash   84

5. Grilled Salmon With Avocado And Bacon Salad   86

6. Chicken And Vegetable Skewers With Peanut Sauce   87

7. Grilled Steak Fajitas With Bell Peppers And

Onions   89

8. Baked Cod With Lemon, Herbs And Zucchini
Noodles   90

9. Low-Carb Meatloaf With Ketchup Glaze And
Roasted Broccoli   92

10. Grilled Chicken Breast With Pesto And
Zucchini Noodles   94

11. Low-Carb Beef And Vegetable Stir-Fry With
Cauliflower Rice   96

12. Baked Salmon With Lemon, Herbs And
Green Beans   98

13. Low-Carb Chicken And Mushroom Creamy
Sauce Over Zucchini Noodles   100

14. Grilled Steak With Roasted Brussels
Sprouts And Sweet Potato   102

15. Low-Carb Chicken And Vegetable Kabobs
With Pesto Sauce   103

Chapter Three   105

Appetizers And Snacks   105

1. Breakfast Scramble With Spinach,
Mushrooms And Goat Cheese   105

2. Low-Carb Protein Smoothie With Banana,
Almond Milk And Chia Seeds   106

3. Low-Carb Cauliflower Fried Rice with Shrimp
and Vegetables   108

4. Baked Salmon And Green Beans   109

5. Low-Carb Chicken And Vegetable Stir-Fry111

6. Prosciutto And Melon Platter   113

7. Italian Delight   114

8. Spanish Delight   115

9. Caprese Skewers   117

10. Gourmet Bites   118

11. Flaxseed Crackers	119
12. Almond Flour Crackers	122
13. Veggie Chips	124
14. Cheese Crisps	126
15. Pork Rinds	128

Soups And Salads — **130**

1. Creamy Tomato Soup	130
2. Chicken And Vegetable Broth	132
3. Cauliflower Soup	134
4. Keto Cream Of Mushroom Soup	136
5. Low-Carb Chicken Noodle Soup	138
6. Spinach And Artichoke Soup	139
7. Roasted Vegetable Soup	141
8. Creamy Asparagus Soup	143
9. Classic Greek Salad	145
10. Spinach And Strawberry Salad	147
11. Keto Cobb Salad	149
12. Low-Carb Chicken Caesar Salad	151
13. Caprese Salad	154
14. Taco Salad	156
15. Chicken And Avocado Salad	158

Entrees — **160**

1. Grilled Steak With Roasted Vegetables	160
2. Beef And Mushroom Stroganoff	162
3. Low-Carb Beef Tacos	164
4. Pork Chop With Apple And Onion	166
5. Cauliflower Fried Rice With Pork	168
6. Chicken And Mushroom Crepes	170
7. Korean-Style Chicken And Vegetable Skewers	171

8. Chicken And Spinach Stuffed Portobellos 173

9. Turkey And Cranberry Meatloaf 175

10. Turkish-Style Stuffed Bell Peppers 177

11. Garlic Shrimp 179

12. Baked Salmon With Lemon And Herbs 181

13. Tuna Steak With Lemon And Herb 183

14. Lobster And Avocado Salad 185

15. Grilled Scallops With Garlic Butter 186

Chapter Four 188

Sides And Vegetables 188

1. Cauliflower Rice And Vegetable Stir-Fry With Broccoli And Bell Peppers 188

2. Zucchini Noodles With Tomato And Mushroom Sauce 190

3. Avocado Toast On Almond Flour Bread With Roasted Brussels Sprouts 192

4. Cauliflower And Mushroom Tacos With Coconut Flour Tortillas 193

5. Cauliflower and Broccoli Cheese Bites On Flaxseed Meal Crackers 194

6. Avocado And Asparagus Bites On Flaxseed Meal Crackers 195

7. Cauliflower And Mushroom Cauliflower Rice Bowl With Coconut Flour Crackers 196

8. Zucchini Noodles With Broccoli And Almond Flour Breadsticks 198

9. Cauliflower Rice And Asparagus With Coconut Flour Tortilla 199

10. Flaxseed Meal Crackers With Avocado And Bell Peppers 200

Desserts 201

1. Keto Cheesecake ... 201
2. Keto Coconut Cream Pie ... 203
3. Keto Pecan Pie ... 205
4. Keto Chocolate Silk Pie ... 207
5. Keto Cheesecake With Almond Flour Crust ... 208
6. Low Carb Cookie Dough Ice Cream ... 210
7. Keto Vanilla Ice Cream ... 212
8. Mason Jar Ice Cream ... 214
9. Dairy-Free Keto Vanilla Ice Cream ... 216
10. 3-Ingredient Keto Ice Cream ... 218

Global Cuisine ... **220**
1. Korean Bibimbap ... 220
2. Indian Butter Chicken ... 222
3. Japanese Teriyaki Salmon ... 224
4. Thai Green Curry ... 225
5. Vietnamese Pho ... 227
6. Chinese Beef And Broccoli ... 229
7. Mexican Carnitas ... 231
8. Greek Gyro ... 233
9. Vietnamese Ceviche ... 235
10. Peruvian Ceviche ... 236

Drinks ... **238**
1. Strawberry Keto Smoothie ... 238
2. Mocha Protein Shake ... 240
3. Blueberry Lemonade Smoothie ... 242
4. Peanut Butter Banana Shake ... 244
5. Pina Colada Protein Smoothie ... 246
6. Vodka Soda ... 248
7. Virgin Mojito ... 250

8. Gin & Tonic 252

9. Cucumber Lime Refresher 254

10. Low-Carb Margarita 256

Chapter Five 258

Meal Planning Tips 258

Grocery Shopping Tips And Tricks 259

Conclusion 261

Tips For Success On A Low-Carb Diet 263

Appendix 265

7-Day Meal Plan 265

Grocery Shopping List And Pantry Staples 266

Conversion Chart 269

Meal Planning Templates 270

Introduction

In today's world, we're constantly bombarded with conflicting messages about what constitutes a "healthy" diet. But one thing is certain: the traditional low-fat, high-carb approach has left many of us feeling unsatisfied, lethargic, and frustrated.

That's why we're thrilled to introduce you to the world of low-carb living, where the focus is on nourishing your body with whole, unprocessed foods that ignite your energy, satisfy your cravings, and support your overall well-being. This cookbook is your passport to a culinary journey that will transform the way you think about food, and more importantly, the way you feel.

For decades, we've been misled by the notion that carbohydrates are the body's primary source of energy. But what if we told you that this isn't entirely true? Your body is capable of adapting to different fuel sources, and when you reduce your carbohydrate intake, your body begins to rely on fat for energy instead. This metabolic state, known as ketosis, is the key to unlocking a wealth of health benefits, from weight loss and improved blood sugar control to increased mental clarity and reduced inflammation.

But don't worry, we're not about deprivation or restriction. We're about empowerment through education and delicious, easy-to-make recipes that will make you wonder how you ever managed without them. From decadent breakfast dishes to satisfying entrees, and from sweet treats to savory snacks, our low-carb cookbook is your ultimate guide to a world of flavor and freedom.

Within these pages, you'll discover:

- How to make mouthwatering low-carb versions of your favorite comfort foods, like pizza, pasta, and bread
- The secret to creating delicious, sugar-free desserts that will satisfy your sweet tooth
- How to make healthy, low-carb swaps for grains, sugars, and processed foods
- Tips and tricks for meal planning, grocery shopping, and cooking like a pro
- The science behind low-carb living, and how it can benefit your overall health
- How to overcome common challenges and stay on track with your low-carb lifestyle
- The importance of listening to your body and making adjustments to your diet as needed

Our recipes are designed to be easy to follow, even for the most novice cooks. We've included a range of options to suit every taste and dietary preference, from vegetarian and vegan to gluten-free and dairy-free. And the best part? You don't have to be a master chef to create these culinary masterpieces. Our recipes are designed to be quick, easy, and accessible to everyone.

So, are you ready to join the low-carb revolution? Are you ready to take control of your health, your energy, and your happiness? Then let's get cooking! In the following pages, we'll show you how to make the most of this incredible way of eating, and how to make delicious, low-carb recipes that will become your new favorites.

Buckle up, friends, and get ready for a culinary adventure that will change your life! With the recipes and knowledge in this cookbook, you'll be empowered to take control of your health and wellbeing, and to live a life that's filled with energy, joy, and delicious food. So let's get started!

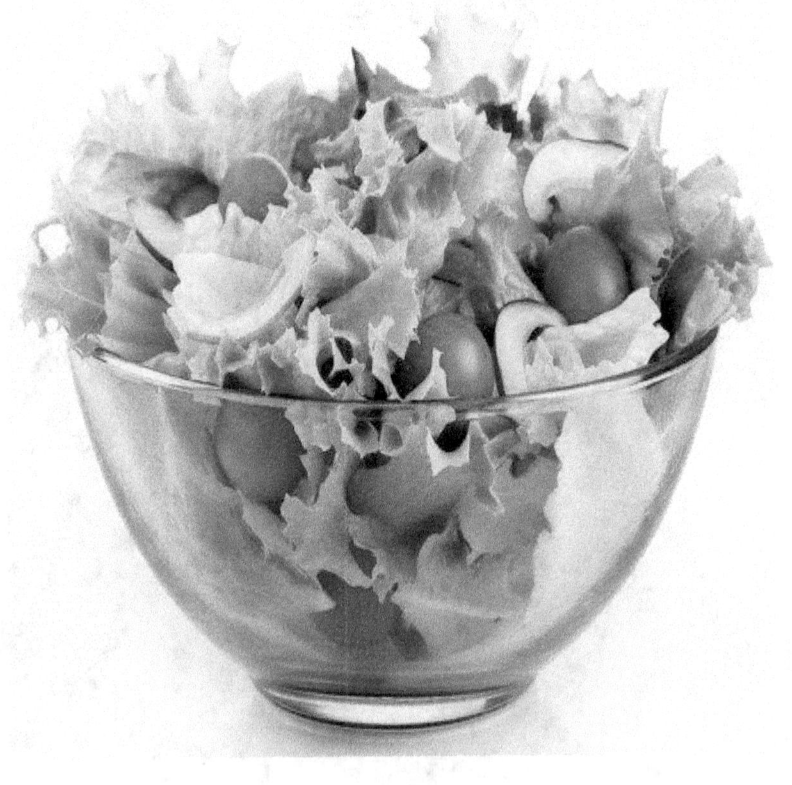

Chapter One

What Is a Low-Carb Diet?

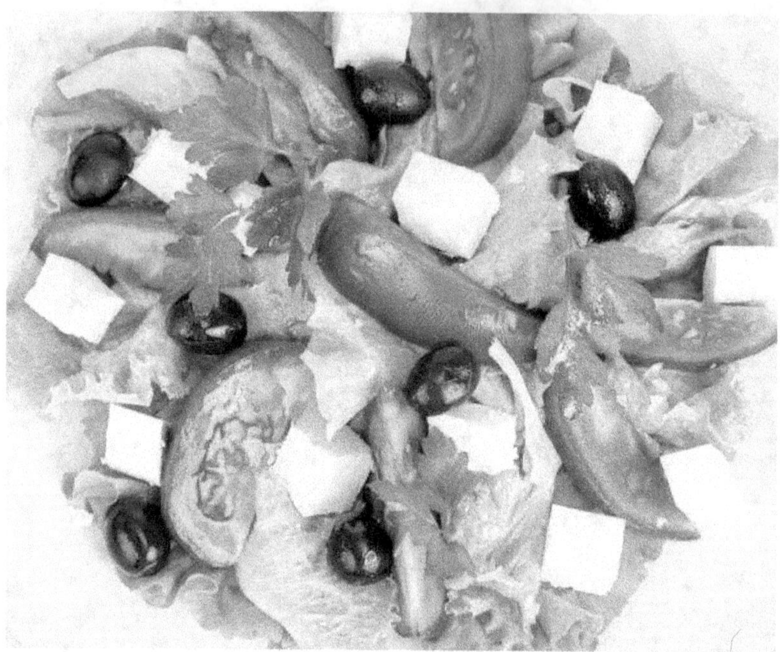

A low-carb diet is an eating plan that restricts the intake of carbohydrates, such as those found in sugary foods, grains, and starchy vegetables. The goal of a low-carb diet is to put the body into a state of ketosis, where it burns fat for energy instead of carbohydrates.

Carbohydrates are the body's primary source of energy, but when we eat too many carbs, our body stores them as glycogen and fat. By reducing our carb intake, we force our body to look for alternative sources of energy, such as fat. This can lead to weight loss, improved blood sugar control, and increased energy levels.

There are different types of low-carb diets, including:

1. Ketogenic Diet (Keto Diet): This diet is very low in carbs (less than 20 grams per day) and high in fat, with moderate protein intake. The goal is to enter a state of ketosis, where the body burns fat for energy.

2. Low-Carb, High-Fat (LCHF) Diet: This diet is similar to the keto diet but allows for more carbs (50-100 grams per day).

3. Atkins Diet: This diet is a low-carb diet that restricts carb intake in phases, starting with a very low-carb phase (20 grams per day) and gradually increasing carb intake.

4. South Beach Diet: This diet is a low-carb diet that restricts carb intake, especially those high in sugar, and emphasizes lean protein and healthy fats.

Foods that are typically restricted on a low-carb diet include:

- Sugary foods: candy, cakes, cookies, and other
sweet treats
- Grains: bread, pasta, rice, and cereals
- Starchy vegetables: potatoes, corn, peas, and
winter squash
- Legumes: beans, lentils, and peanuts
- Fruit: some fruits, such as bananas and apples,
are high in carbs and may be restricted

**Foods that are typically encouraged on a
low-carb diet include:**

- Meat: beef, pork, lamb, and chicken
- Fish and seafood: salmon, tuna, shrimp, and
lobster
- Eggs
- Full-fat dairy: cheese, butter, and cream
- Vegetables: leafy greens, broccoli, cauliflower,
and avocado
- Nuts and seeds: almonds, walnuts, chia seeds,
and flax seeds
- Healthy oils: olive oil, coconut oil, and avocado oil

Benefits Of A Low-Carb LifeStyle

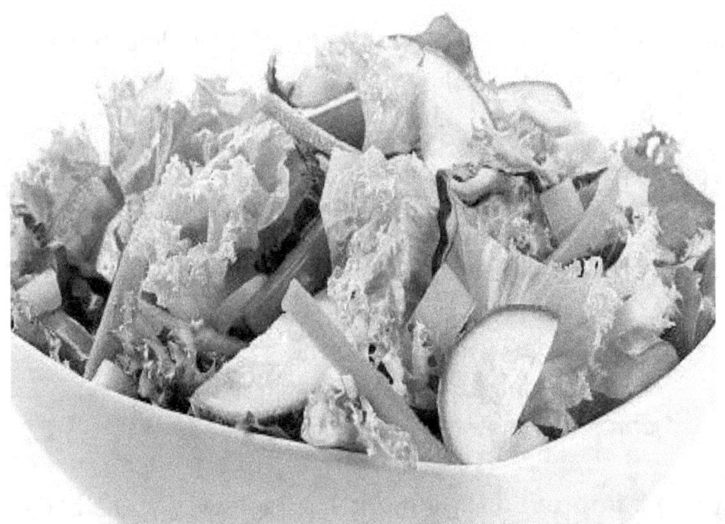

A low-carb lifestyle has numerous benefits, including:

1. Weight Loss: Reducing carbohydrate intake leads to weight loss, as it forces the body to burn stored fat for energy.

2. Improved Blood Sugar Control: Low-carb diets help regulate blood sugar levels and improve insulin sensitivity, reducing the risk of developing type 2 diabetes.

3. Increased Energy: The high-fat diet associated with low-carb living provides a sustained energy source, reducing the need for carbohydrates.

4. Reduced Triglycerides: Low-carb diets have been shown to decrease triglyceride levels, a risk factor for heart disease.

5. Improved Mental Clarity: Many individuals report improved focus and mental clarity when following a low-carb lifestyle.

6. Reduced Inflammation: Low-carb diets have anti-inflammatory effects, which may help with chronic pain and inflammation.

7. Improved Digestion: The high-fat, low-carb diet can improve digestion and reduce symptoms of irritable bowel syndrome (IBS).

8. Reduced Acne: Some individuals report improved skin health and reduced acne when following a low-carb lifestyle.

9. Improved Heart Health: Low-carb diets may help lower blood pressure, improve HDL cholesterol levels, and reduce the risk of heart disease.

10. Reduced Cancer Risk: Some research suggests that low-carb diets may help reduce the risk of certain cancers, such as colon, breast, and prostate cancer.

11. Improved Dental Health: The reduced sugar intake associated with low-carb living can help prevent tooth decay and improve oral health.

12. Reduced Migraines: Some individuals report a reduction in migraine frequency and severity when following a low-carb lifestyle.

13. Improved Immune Function: Low-carb diets may help boost the immune system, reducing the risk of illnesses like the common cold and flu.

14. Reduced Anxiety and Depression: Some individuals report improved mental health and reduced symptoms of anxiety and depression when following a low-carb lifestyle.

15. Increased Human Growth Hormone (HGH) Production: Low-carb diets have been shown to increase production of HGH, which can help with weight loss and muscle gain.

Understanding Net Carbs

Net carbs are the total carbohydrate content of a food or meal minus its fiber and sugar alcohol content. The concept of net carbs is popular among low-carb dieters, as it helps them focus on the carbohydrates that are most likely to impact their blood sugar levels and weight management.

The formula to calculate net carbs is:

Net Carbs = Total Carbohydrates - Fiber - Sugar Alcohols

Here's a breakdown of each component:

1. Total Carbohydrates: This includes all the carbs in a food or meal, including sugars, starches, and fiber.

2. Fiber: This is a type of carbohydrate that is not digestible by the body and does not raise blood sugar levels. Fiber is subtracted from the total carbohydrate count because it does not contribute to the overall carb content.

3. Sugar Alcohols: These are sweeteners like xylitol, erythritol, and sorbitol that are low in calories and do not raise blood sugar levels. They are also subtracted from the total carbohydrate count.

For example, let's say a food label shows:

- Total Carbohydrates: 20g
- Fiber: 5g
- Sugar Alcohols: 3g

To calculate the net carbs, you would subtract the fiber and sugar alcohols from the total carbohydrates:

Net Carbs = 20g - 5g - 3g = 12g

This means that the food contains 12g of net carbs, which is the amount that will impact blood sugar levels and weight management.

Understanding net carbs is important for people following a low-carb diet, as it helps them make informed choices about the foods they eat. However, it's important to note that the concept of net carbs is not universally accepted, and some experts argue that it can be misleading. Always consult with a healthcare professional or registered dietitian for personalized nutrition advice.

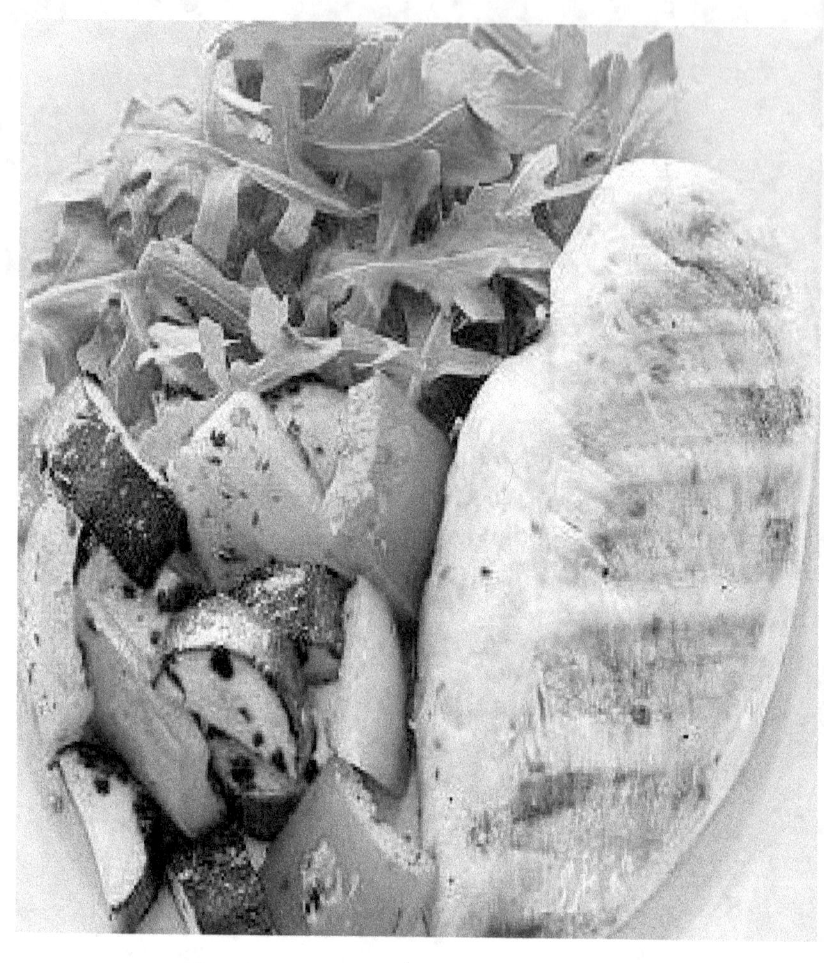

Chapter Two

Mouth-Watering Breakfast Recipes

1. Spinach And Feta Omelette

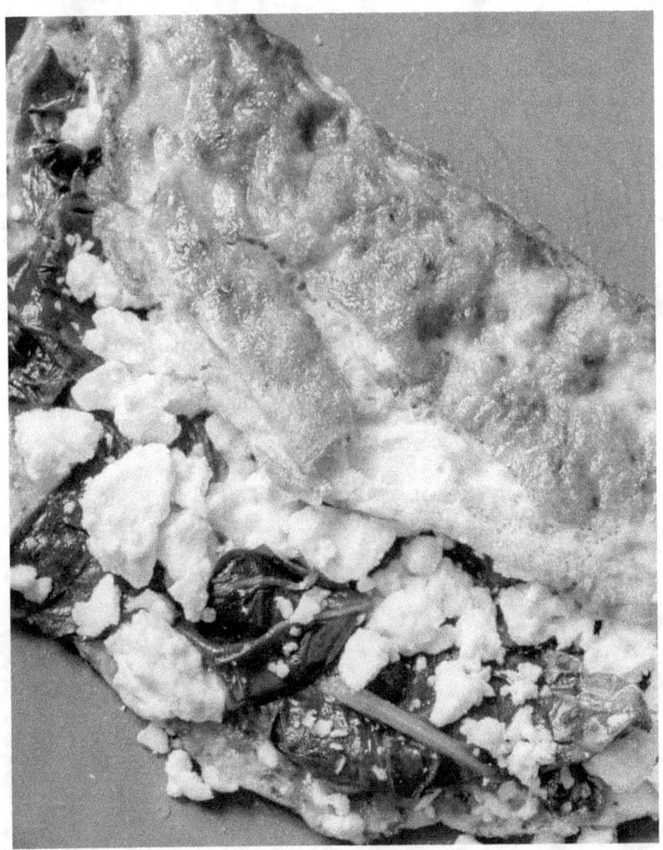

Ingredients:
- 2 large eggs
- 1/4 cup chopped fresh spinach
- 1/4 cup crumbled feta cheese
- 1/2 teaspoon garlic powder
- Salt and pepper to taste
- 1 tablespoon butter or oil

Instructions:
1. In a small bowl, beat the eggs and set aside.
2. Heat a medium non-stick skillet over medium heat. Add butter or oil and melt.
3. Add the chopped spinach and cook until wilted, about 1-2 minutes.
4. Pour the beaten eggs over the spinach and cook until the edges start to set.
5. Sprinkle the crumbled feta cheese over the eggs.
6. Use a spatula to gently fold the omelet in half.
7. Cook for another minute, until the cheese is melted and the eggs are cooked through.
8. Serve hot and enjoy!

This recipe has approximately 320 calories, 22g protein, 24g fat, and only 4g net carbs. The spinach and feta add a delicious flavor and texture combination that's perfect for a low-carb breakfast.

2. Mushroom And Cheddar Scrambled Eggs

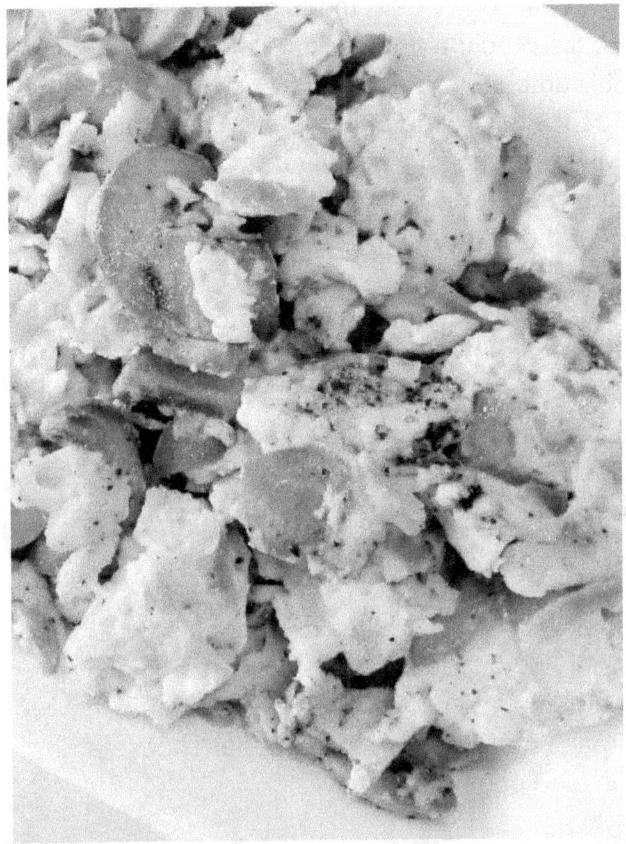

Ingredients:
- 2 large eggs
- 1/2 cup sliced mushrooms (button, cremini, or shiitake)
- 1/4 cup shredded cheddar cheese
- 1/2 teaspoon dried thyme
- Salt and pepper to taste

- 1 tablespoon butter or oil

Instructions:
1. In a small bowl, beat the eggs and set aside.
2. Heat a medium non-stick skillet over medium heat. Add butter or oil and melt.
3. Add the sliced mushrooms and cook until they release their moisture and start to brown, about 3-4 minutes.
4. Pour the beaten eggs over the mushrooms and cook until the eggs start to set.
5. Sprinkle the shredded cheddar cheese over the eggs and add thyme.
6. Use a spatula to gently scramble the eggs, breaking them up into small curds.
7. Cook for another minute, until the cheese is melted and the eggs are cooked through.
8. Serve hot and enjoy!

This recipe has approximately 340 calories, 20g protein, 26g fat, and only 4g net carbs. The mushrooms add a meaty texture and earthy flavor that pairs perfectly with the cheddar cheese and scrambled eggs.

3. Smoked Salmon And Cream Cheese Omelette

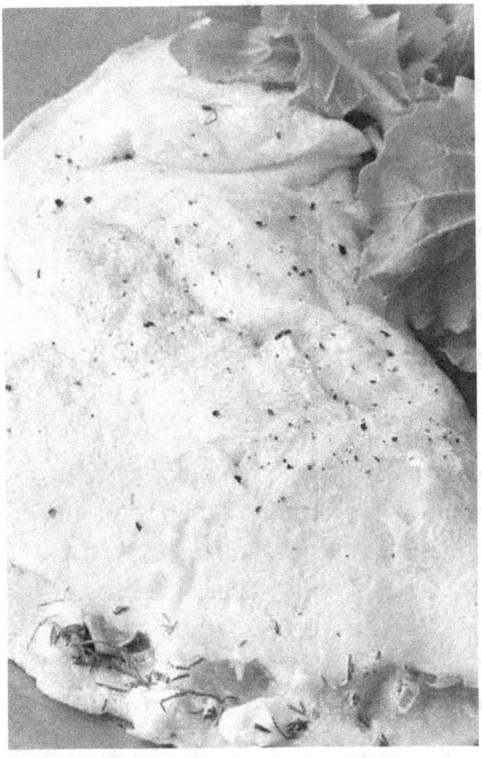

Ingredients:

- 2 large eggs
- 2 slices smoked salmon (about 2 ounces)
- 1 tablespoon cream cheese, softened
- 1/4 cup chopped fresh dill
- Salt and pepper to taste
- 1 tablespoon butter or oil

Instructions:

1. In a small bowl, beat the eggs and set aside.
2. Heat a medium non-stick skillet over medium heat. Add butter or oil and melt.
3. Add the chopped fresh dill and cook for 1 minute, until fragrant.
4. Add the slices of smoked salmon and cook for 1-2 minutes, until heated through.
5. Pour the beaten eggs over the salmon and dill.
6. Dollop the softened cream cheese on top of the eggs.
7. Use a spatula to gently fold the omelet in half.
8. Cook for another minute, until the eggs are cooked through and the cheese is melted.
9. Serve hot and enjoy!

This recipe has approximately 360 calories, 22g protein, 28g fat, and only 4g net carbs. The smoked salmon adds a rich, savory flavor and a boost of omega-3 fatty acids, while the cream cheese adds a tangy creaminess. The fresh dill adds a bright, fresh note to the dish.

4. Bacon And Spinach Scrambled Eggs

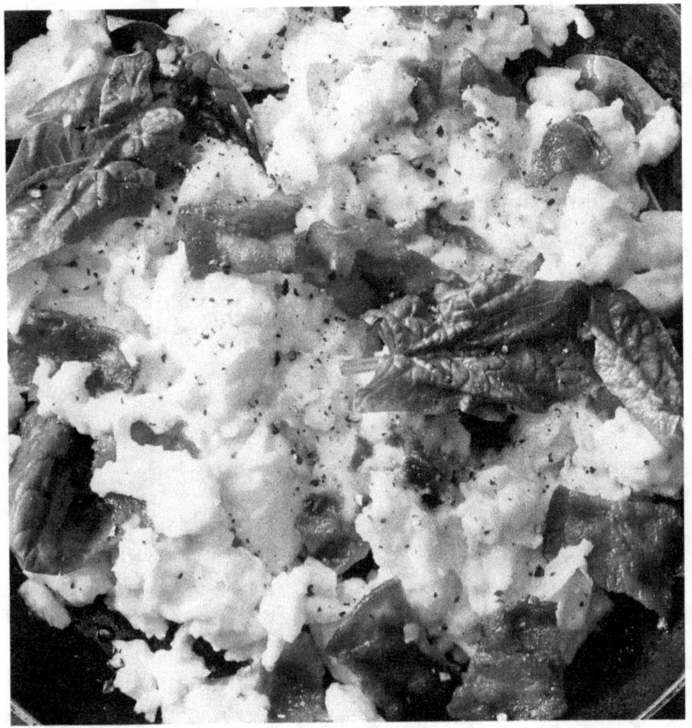

Ingredients:

- 2 large eggs
- 2 slices cooked bacon, crumbled
- 1/2 cup chopped fresh spinach
- 1/2 teaspoon garlic powder
- Salt and pepper to taste
- 1 tablespoon butter or oil

Instructions:

1. In a small bowl, beat the eggs and set aside.

2. Heat a medium non-stick skillet over medium
heat. Add butter or oil and melt.
3. Add the crumbled bacon and cook for 1 minute,
until fragrant.
4. Add the chopped spinach and cook until wilted,
about 1-2 minutes.
5. Pour the beaten eggs over the bacon and
spinach.
6. Sprinkle the garlic powder over the eggs.
7. Use a spatula to gently scramble the eggs,
breaking them up into small curds.
8. Cook for another minute, until the eggs are
cooked through.
9. Serve hot and enjoy.

This recipe has approximately 320 calories, 20g
protein, 24g fat, and only 4g net carbs. The bacon
adds a smoky, savory flavor, while the spinach
adds a boost of nutrients and flavor. The garlic
powder adds a subtle depth to the dish.

5. Caprese Omelette

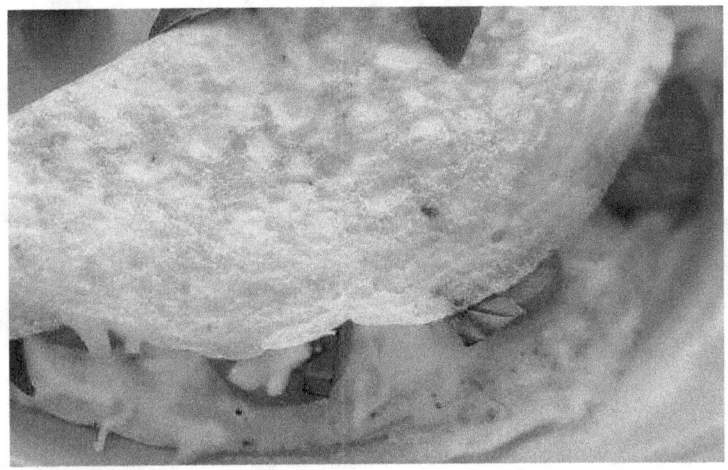

Ingredients:
- 2 large eggs
- 1/4 cup sliced fresh mozzarella cheese
- 1/4 cup sliced fresh tomatoes
- 1/4 cup chopped fresh basil
- Salt and pepper to taste
- 1 tablespoon butter or oil

Instructions:
1. In a small bowl, beat the eggs and set aside.
2. Heat a medium non-stick skillet over medium heat. Add butter or oil and melt.
3. Add the sliced mozzarella cheese and cook for 1 minute, until melted.
4. Add the sliced tomatoes and cook for another minute.
5. Pour the beaten eggs over the cheese and tomatoes.

6. Sprinkle the chopped basil over the eggs.
7. Use a spatula to gently fold the omelet in half.
8. Cook for another minute, until the eggs are cooked through.
9. Serve hot and enjoy.

This recipe has approximately 300 calories, 18g protein, 22g fat, and only 4g net carbs. The fresh mozzarella, tomatoes, and basil create a flavorful and colorful omelet that's perfect for a low-carb breakfast.

6. Almond Flour Pancakes

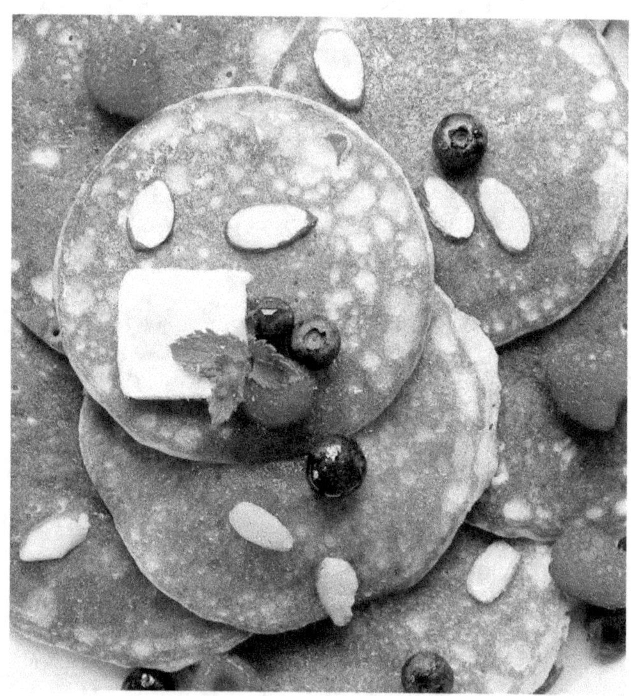

Ingredients:
- 1 1/2 cups almond flour
- 3 large eggs
- 1/2 cup unsweetened almond milk
- 1/4 cup melted coconut oil
- 1/2 teaspoon vanilla extract
- Pinch of salt

Instructions:
1. In a large bowl, combine almond flour, eggs, almond milk, melted coconut oil, vanilla extract, and salt. Mix well until smooth.
2. Heat a non-stick skillet or griddle over medium heat.
3. Drop batter by 1/4 cupfuls onto the skillet or griddle.
4. Cook for 2-3 minutes or until bubbles appear on the surface and edges start to dry.
5. Flip and cook for another 1-2 minutes or until golden brown.
6. Serve warm with your favorite toppings, such as butter, sugar-free syrup, fresh berries, or whipped cream.

Tips:
- Make sure to use blanched almond flour for the best texture.
- Adjust the amount of almond milk to achieve the desired consistency.
- Keep the pancakes small to ensure they cook evenly.

Nutritional information (per serving):

- Calories: 320
- Protein: 6g
- Fat: 26g
- Carbohydrates: 5g
- Fiber: 2g
- Net Carbs: 3g

7. Coconut Flour Waffles

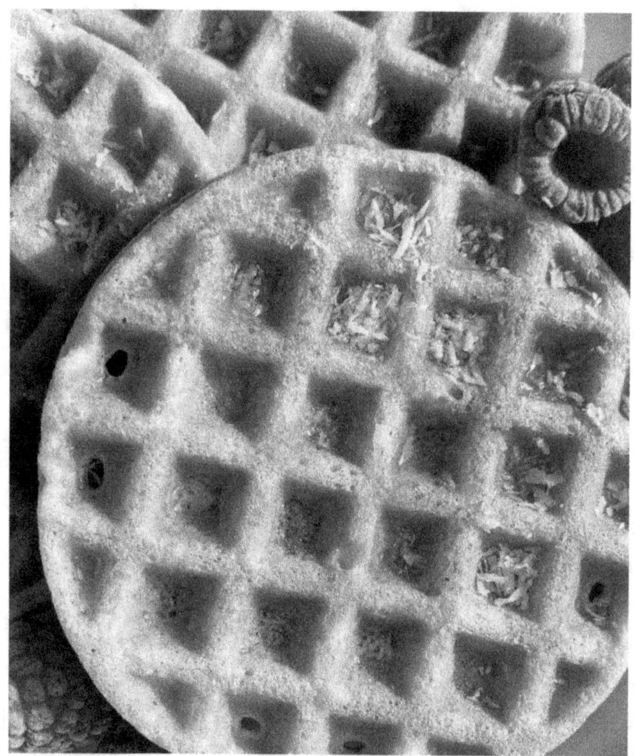

Ingredients:

- 1 cup coconut flour
- 4 large eggs
- 1/2 cup unsweetened coconut milk
- 1/4 cup melted coconut oil
- 1/2 teaspoon vanilla extract
- Pinch of salt

Instructions:
1. Preheat your waffle iron according to the manufacturer's instructions.
2. In a large bowl, combine coconut flour, eggs, coconut milk, melted coconut oil, vanilla extract, and salt. Mix well until smooth.
3. The batter should still be slightly lumpy.
4. Pour about 1/4 cup of the batter onto the center of the waffle iron.
5. Close the iron and cook for 3-5 minutes or until the waffles are golden brown and crispy.
6. Repeat with the remaining batter, greasing the waffle iron with coconut oil or cooking spray as needed.
7. Serve warm with your favorite toppings, such as butter, sugar-free syrup, fresh berries, or whipped cream.

Tips:
- Make sure to use a high-quality coconut flour that is finely ground.
- Adjust the amount of coconut milk to achieve the desired consistency.
- Keep the waffles small to ensure they cook evenly.

Nutritional information (per serving):
- Calories: 350
- Protein: 6g
- Fat: 28g
- Carbohydrates: 5g
- Fiber: 3g
- Net Carbs: 2g

8. Cream Cheese Pancakes

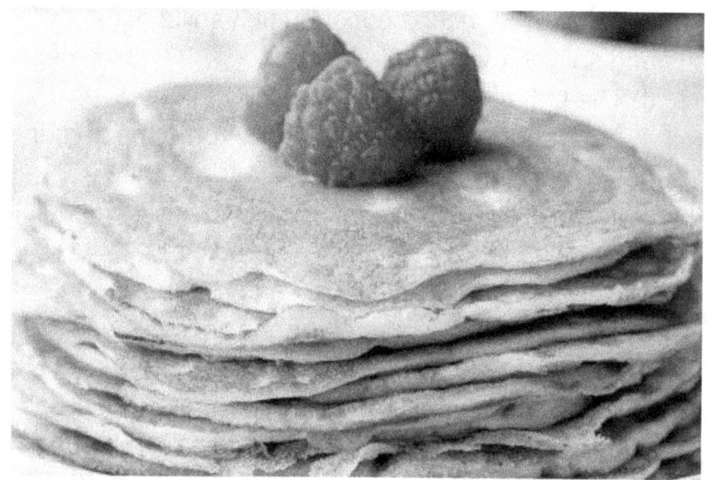

Ingredients:
- 1 1/2 cups almond flour
- 3 large eggs
- 1/2 cup unsweetened almond milk
- 1/4 cup softened cream cheese
- 1/2 teaspoon vanilla extract
- Pinch of salt

Instructions:
1. In a large bowl, combine almond flour, eggs, almond milk, softened cream cheese, vanilla extract, and salt. Mix well until smooth.
2. Heat a non-stick skillet or griddle over medium heat.
3. Drop batter by 1/4 cupfuls onto the skillet or griddle.
4. Cook for 2-3 minutes or until bubbles appear on the surface and edges start to dry.
5. Flip and cook for another 1-2 minutes or until golden brown.
6. Serve warm with your favorite toppings, such as butter, sugar-free syrup, fresh berries, or whipped cream.

Tips:
- Make sure to use a high-quality cream cheese that is softened to room temperature.
- Adjust the amount of almond milk to achieve the desired consistency.
- Keep the pancakes small to ensure they cook evenly.

Nutritional information (per serving):
- Calories: 340
- Protein: 7g
- Fat: 28g
- Carbohydrates: 5g
- Fiber: 2g
- Net Carbs: 3g

9. Keto Cinnamon Roll Waffles

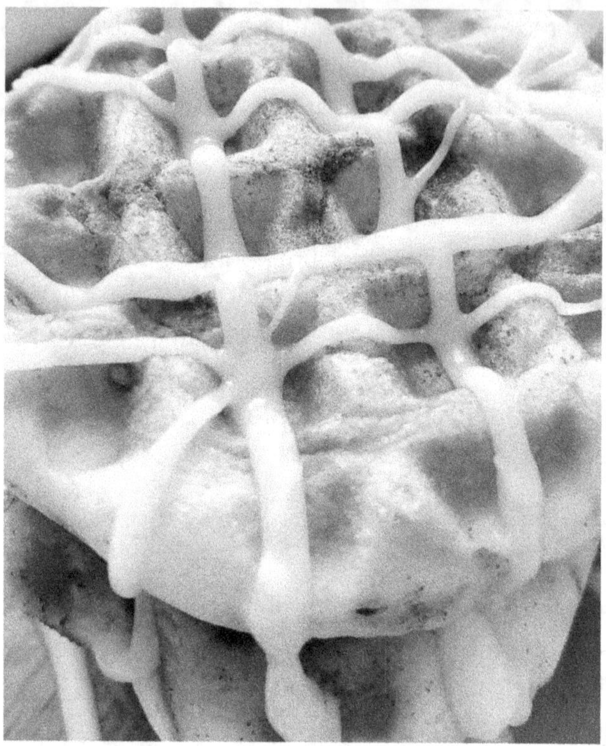

Ingredients:
- 1 cup almond flour
- 4 large eggs
- 1/2 cup unsweetened almond milk
- 1/4 cup melted coconut oil
- 1/2 teaspoon ground cinnamon
- 1/4 teaspoon ground nutmeg
- Pinch of salt

Instructions:

1. Preheat your waffle iron according to the manufacturer's instructions.
2. In a large bowl, combine almond flour, eggs, almond milk, melted coconut oil, cinnamon, nutmeg, and salt. Mix well until smooth.
3. Pour about 1/4 cup of the batter onto the center of the waffle iron.
4. Close the iron and cook for 3-5 minutes or until the waffles are golden brown and crispy.
5. Repeat with the remaining batter, greasing the waffle iron with coconut oil or cooking spray as needed.
6. Serve warm with your favorite toppings, such as butter, sugar-free syrup, fresh berries, or whipped cream.

Tips:
- Make sure to use a high-quality almond flour that is finely ground.
- Adjust the amount of almond milk to achieve the desired consistency.
- Keep the waffles small to ensure they cook evenly.

Nutritional information (per serving):
- Calories: 360
- Protein: 7g
- Fat: 30g
- Carbohydrates: 5g
- Fiber: 3g
- Net Carbs: 2g

10. Lemon Ricotta Pancakes

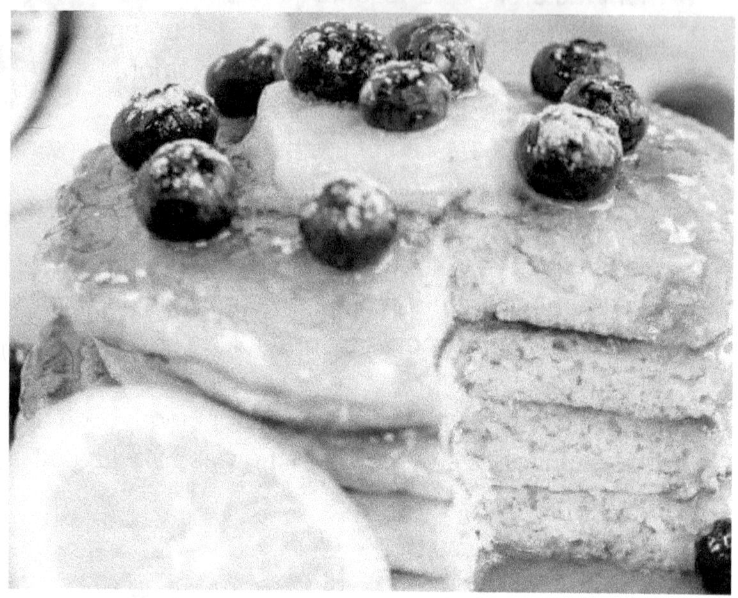

Ingredients:

- 1 1/2 cups almond flour
- 3 large eggs
- 1/2 cup unsweetened almond milk
- 1/4 cup ricotta cheese
- 1 tablespoon freshly squeezed lemon juice
- 1/2 teaspoon vanilla extract
- Pinch of salt

Instructions:

1. In a large bowl, combine almond flour, eggs, almond milk, ricotta cheese, lemon juice, vanilla extract, and salt. Mix well until smooth.
2. Heat a non-stick skillet or griddle over medium heat.

3. Drop batter by 1/4 cupfuls onto the skillet or griddle.
4. Cook for 2-3 minutes or until bubbles appear on the surface and edges start to dry.
5. Flip and cook for another 1-2 minutes or until golden brown.
6. Serve warm with your favorite toppings, such as butter, sugar-free syrup, fresh berries, or whipped cream.

Tips:
- Make sure to use high-quality ricotta cheese that is full-fat.
- Adjust the amount of almond milk to achieve the desired consistency.
- Keep the pancakes small to ensure they cook evenly.

Nutritional information (per serving):
- Calories: 330
- Protein: 8g
- Fat: 26g
- Carbohydrates: 5g
- Fiber: 2g
- Net Carbs: 3g

11. Sugar-Free Maple Bacon

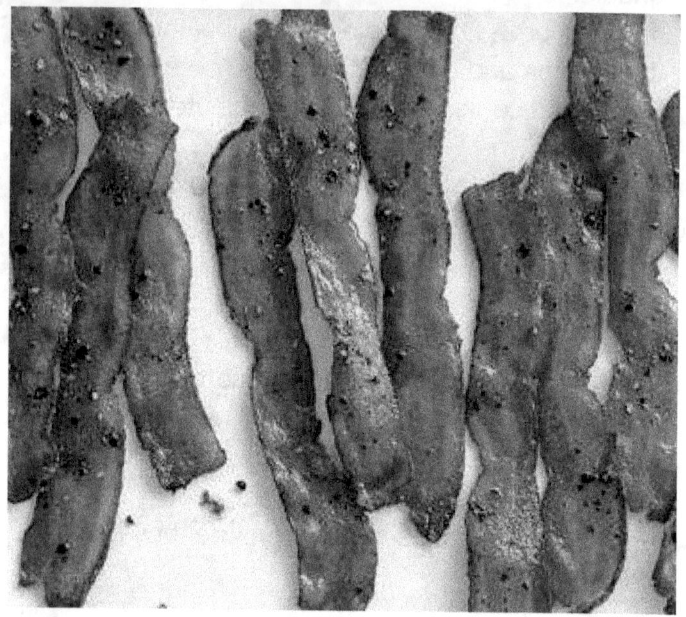

Ingredients:
- 12 slices of bacon
- 1/4 cup sugar-free maple syrup (made with stevia or erythritol)
- 1/2 teaspoon black pepper

Instructions:
1. Preheat the oven to 400°F (200°C).
2. Line a baking sheet with aluminum foil or parchment paper.
3. Lay the bacon slices on the prepared baking sheet.
4. Drizzle the sugar-free maple syrup evenly over the bacon slices.

5. Sprinkle black pepper to taste.
6. Bake for 20-25 minutes or until crispy and golden brown.
7. Remove from the oven and let cool completely.

This recipe yields 12 slices of delicious sugar-free maple bacon, perfect for a low-carb breakfast.

12. Low-Carb Breakfast Sausage

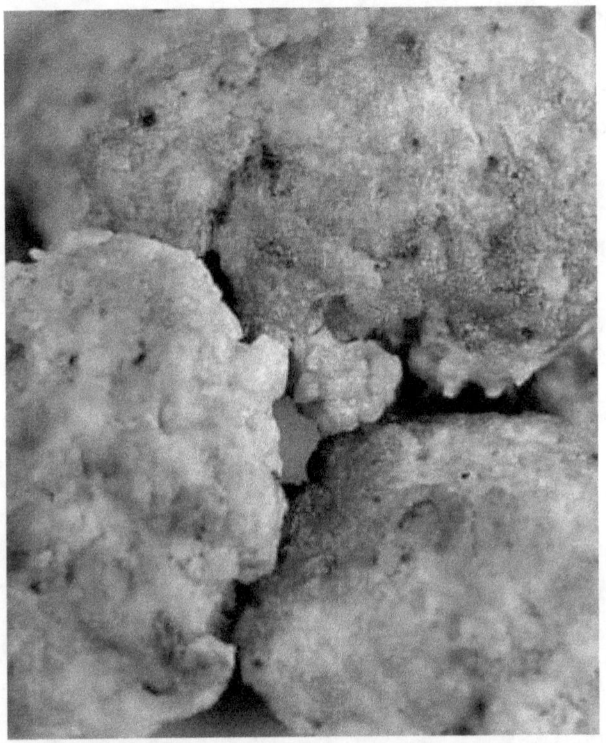

Ingredients:
- 1 pound ground sausage meat (made with pork, chicken, or turkey)

- 1/2 cup almond flour
- 1/4 cup grated cheddar cheese
- 1 egg
- 1/2 teaspoon salt
- 1/4 teaspoon black pepper
- 1/4 teaspoon sage

Instructions:
1. Preheat a skillet over medium-high heat.
2. In a large bowl, combine sausage meat, almond flour, cheese, egg, salt, pepper, and sage. Mix well with your hands or a wooden spoon until just combined.
3. Form into 4-6 patties, depending on desired size.
4. Add the patties to the skillet and cook for 4-5 minutes per side, or until cooked through.
5. Serve hot and enjoy.

13. Low-Carb Ham Steak

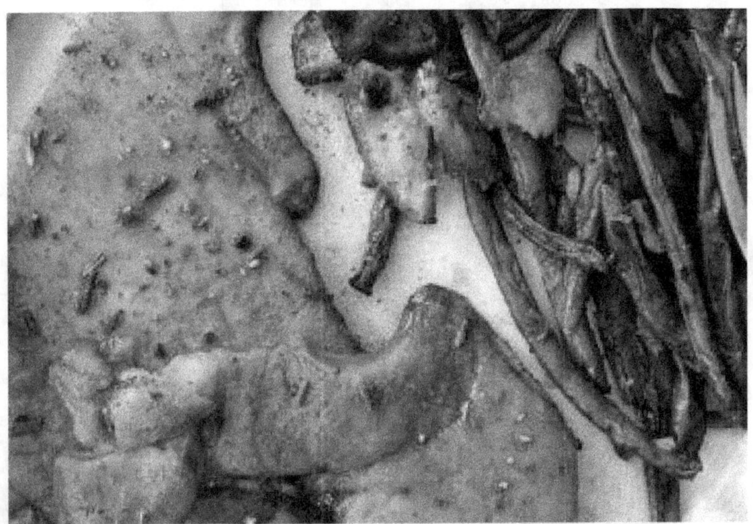

Ingredients:
- 1 (6-ounce) ham steak
- 1/4 cup sugar-free glaze (made with stevia or erythritol)
- 1/4 cup pineapple juice (optional)

Instructions:
1. Preheat a skillet or grill over medium heat.
2. In a small bowl, mix together the sugar-free glaze and pineapple juice (if using).
3. Brush the glaze mixture evenly over both sides of the ham steak.
4. Add the ham steak to the skillet or grill and cook for 4-5 minutes per side, or until caramelized and cooked through.
5. Serve hot and enjoy.

This recipe yields 1 delicious low-carb ham steak, perfect for breakfast. You can also serve it with a side of roasted vegetables or a low-carb breakfast side dish.

14. Low-Carb Canadian Bacon

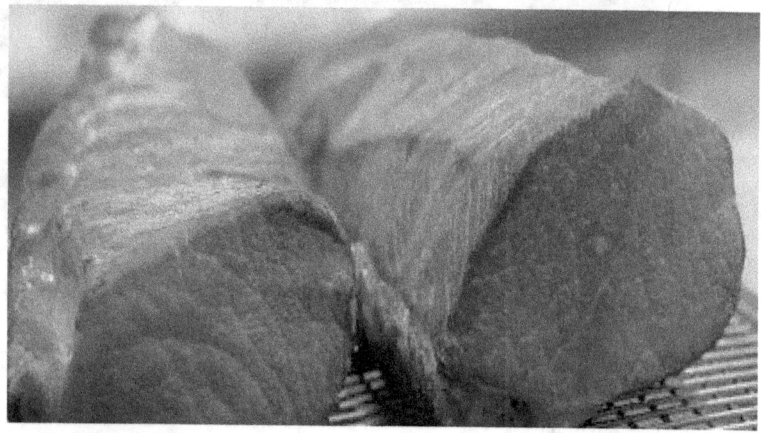

Ingredients:
- 4 slices of Canadian bacon
- 1/4 cup sugar-free maple syrup (made with stevia or erythritol)
- 1/4 teaspoon black pepper

Instructions:
1. Preheat the oven to 400°F (200°C).
2. Line a baking sheet with aluminum foil or parchment paper.
3. Lay the Canadian bacon slices on the prepared baking sheet.

4. Drizzle the sugar-free maple syrup evenly over the Canadian bacon slices.

5. Sprinkle black pepper to taste.

6. Bake for 15-20 minutes or until crispy and golden brown.

7. Remove from the oven and let cool completely.

This recipe yields 4 slices of delicious low-carb Canadian bacon, perfect for a breakfast. You can also use it in low-carb breakfast sandwiches or wraps.

15. Low-Carb Steak And Eggs

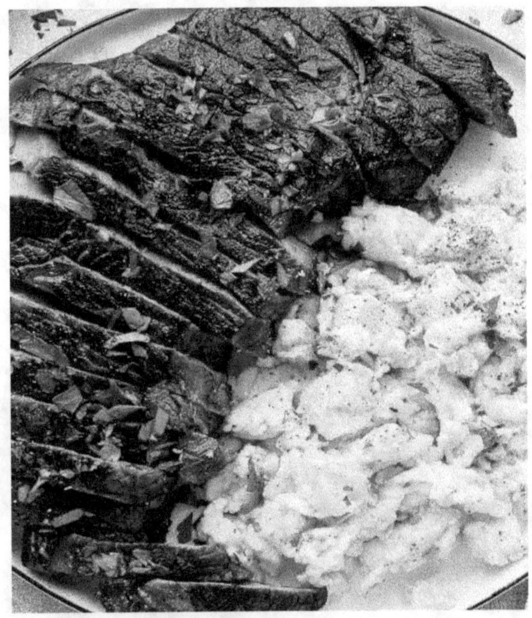

Ingredients:
- 1.5 pounds ribeye or strip steak

- 4 eggs
- 1/4 cup cheese (optional)
- 1/4 cup spinach (optional)
- Salt and pepper to taste

Instructions:
1. Preheat a skillet or grill over medium-high heat.
2. Season the steak with salt and pepper.
3. Add the steak to the skillet or grill and cook for 4-5 minutes per side, or until cooked to desired doneness.
4. While the steak is cooking, fry the eggs in a separate skillet.
5. Serve the steak with the fried eggs, cheese, and spinach (if using).
6. Enjoy your delicious low-carb steak and eggs!

This recipe yields 1 steak and 4 eggs, perfect for a hearty low-carb breakfast. You can also customize it with your favorite cheese and vegetables.

Delicious Lunch Recipes

1. Grilled Chicken Breast With Avocado Salad

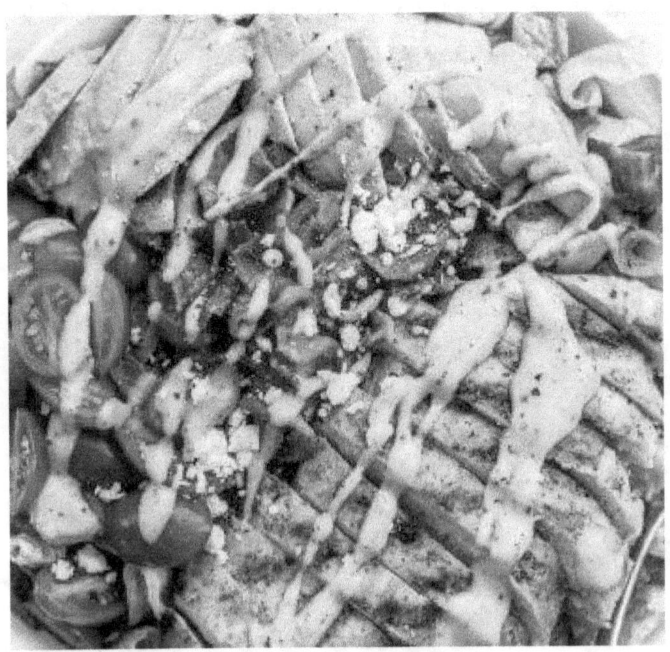

Ingredients:
- 4 boneless, skinless chicken breasts
- 2 ripe avocados, diced
- 1/2 cup mixed greens
- 1/4 cup cherry tomatoes, halved
- 1/4 cup sliced red onion
- 2 tbsp olive oil
- 1 tbsp lemon juice
- Salt and pepper to taste

Instructions:
1. Preheat the grill to medium-high heat.
2. Season chicken breasts with salt and pepper.
3. Grill chicken for 5-6 minutes per side, or until cooked through.
4. In a large bowl, combine mixed greens, avocado, cherry tomatoes, and red onion.
5. Slice grilled chicken and add to salad.
6. Drizzle with olive oil and lemon juice.
7. Serve immediately and enjoy!

This recipe yields 4 servings, with approximately 350 calories, 30g protein, 25g fat, and 5g net carbs per serving.

2. Low-Carb Turkey Lettuce Wraps

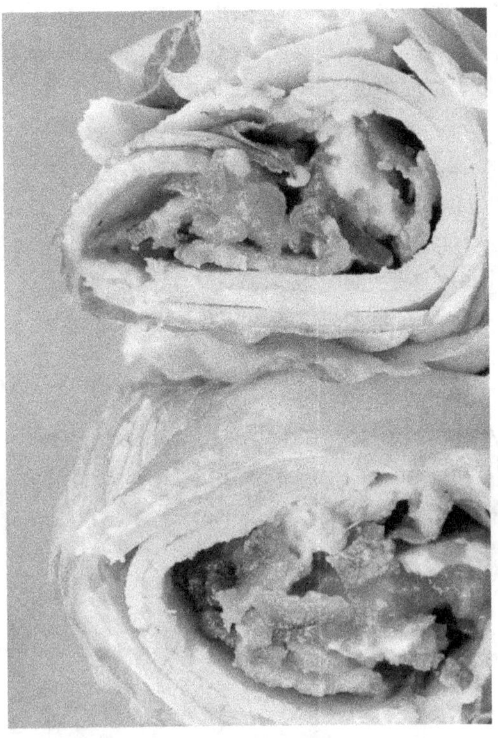

Ingredients:

- 4 slices of deli turkey breast
- 4 lettuce leaves
- 1/4 cup sliced avocado
- 1/4 cup sliced tomato
- 1/4 cup sliced bacon
- 2 tbsp mayonnaise
- 1 tsp Dijon mustard (optional)

Instructions:

1. Lay lettuce leaves flat on a clean surface.
2. Arrange 1 slice of turkey breast on each lettuce leaf.
3. Add sliced avocado, tomato, and bacon on top of the turkey.
4. Drizzle with mayonnaise and Dijon mustard (if using).
5. Fold lettuce leaves to enclose filling.
6. Serve immediately and enjoy!

This recipe yields 4 servings, with approximately 350 calories, 30g protein, 25g fat, and 5g net carbs per serving.

By the way, you can also customize this recipe with other low-carb ingredients like cheese, spinach, or bell peppers. Just remember to keep the carb count in mind.

3. Tuna Salad With Celery Sticks

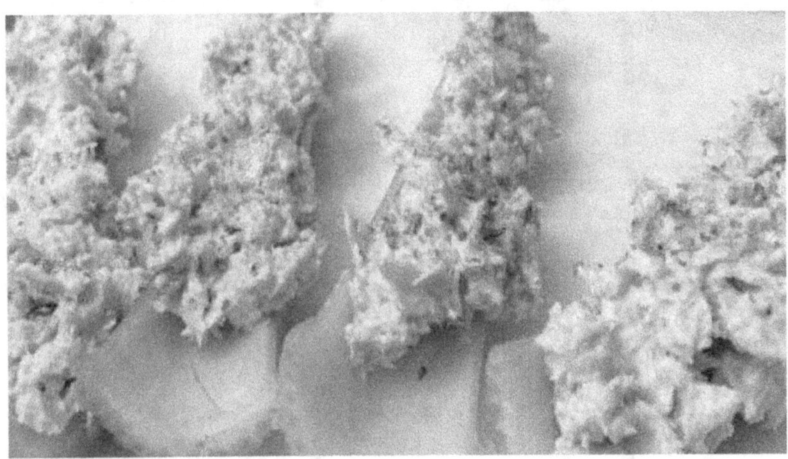

Ingredients:
- 1 can of tuna (drained and flaked)
- 1/4 cup mayonnaise
- 1/4 cup chopped celery
- 1/4 cup chopped red onion
- 1/4 cup chopped hard-boiled egg
- Salt and pepper to taste
- 4 celery sticks

Instructions:
1. In a medium bowl, combine tuna, mayonnaise, celery, onion, and egg.
2. Mix well until all ingredients are fully incorporated.
3. Season with salt and pepper to taste.
4. Cover and refrigerate for at least 30 minutes to allow flavors to meld.
5. Serve tuna salad on celery sticks.

This recipe yields 4 servings, with approximately 250 calories, 30g protein, 15g fat, and 5g net carbs per serving.

You can also customize this recipe with other low-carb ingredients like diced bell peppers or avocado. Just remember to keep the carb count in mind.

4. Zucchini Boats With Turkey And Cheese

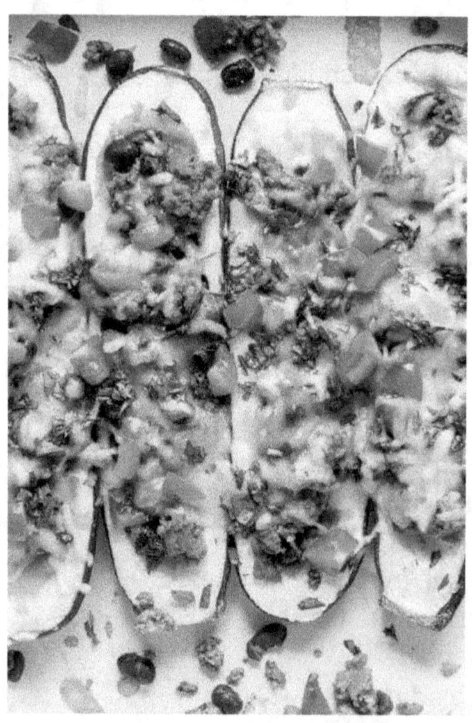

Ingredients:
- 4 medium zucchinis
- 4 slices of deli turkey breast
- 1/4 cup shredded cheddar cheese
- 1/4 cup chopped fresh parsley
- 2 tbsp olive oil
- Salt and pepper to taste

Instructions:
1. Preheat the oven to 375°F (190°C).
2. Cut zucchinis in half lengthwise and scoop out the insides.
3. Arrange zucchinis on a baking sheet lined with parchment paper.
4. Divide turkey slices among zucchinis, placing them inside the hollowed-out centers.
5. Sprinkle shredded cheese over turkey.
6. Drizzle with olive oil and sprinkle with parsley.
7. Season with salt and pepper to taste.
8. Bake for 20-25 minutes or until zucchinis are tender.

This recipe yields 4 servings, with approximately 250 calories, 30g protein, 15g fat, and 5g net carbs per serving.

5. Cauliflower Fried Rice With Shrimp

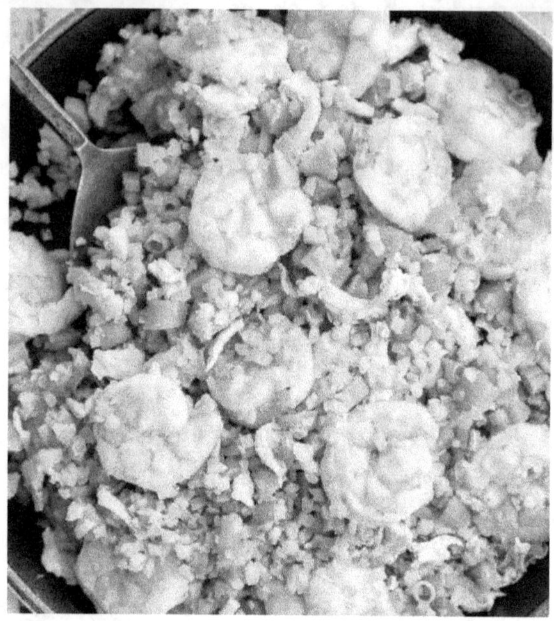

Ingredients:
- 1 head of cauliflower
- 1 cup cooked shrimp
- 2 tbsp coconut oil
- 1 small onion, diced
- 2 cloves garlic, minced
- 1 cup mixed vegetables (e.g., peas, carrots, corn)
- 2 tbsp soy sauce
- 1 tsp oyster sauce (optional)
- Salt and pepper to taste

Instructions:

1. Pulse cauliflower in a food processor until it resembles rice.
2. Heat coconut oil in a large skillet or wok over medium-high heat.
3. Add onion and garlic and cook until softened.
4. Add mixed vegetables and cook until tender.
5. Add cooked shrimp and stir to combine.
6. Add cauliflower "rice" and stir-fry until combined with vegetables and shrimp.
7. Add soy sauce and oyster sauce (if using) and season with salt and pepper.
8. Serve immediately.

This recipe yields 4 servings, with approximately 250 calories, 20g protein, 15g fat, and 5g net carbs per serving.

6. Keto Cobb Salad

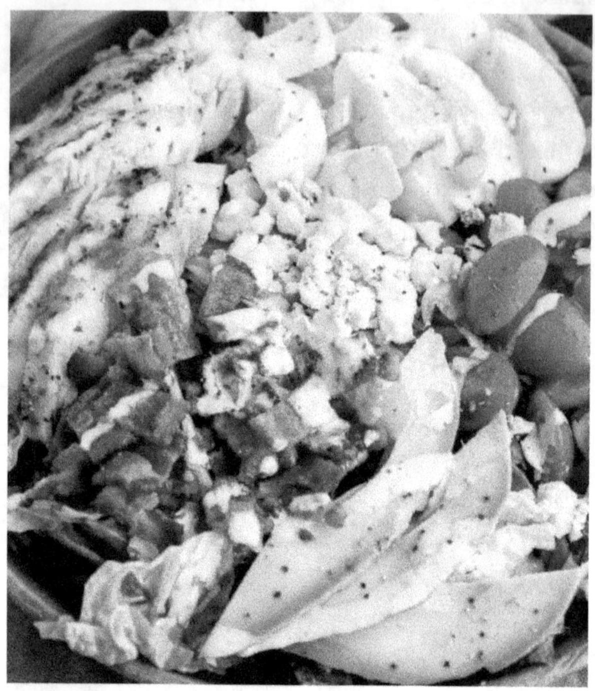

Ingredients:
- 4 cups mixed greens
- 1 cup cooked chicken breast, diced
- 1/2 cup diced avocado
- 1/2 cup diced bacon
- 1/4 cup diced red onion
- 1/4 cup diced hard-boiled egg
- 1/4 cup chopped fresh chives
- 2 tbsp olive oil
- 1 tbsp lemon juice
- Salt and pepper to taste

Instructions:
1. In a large bowl, combine mixed greens, chicken breast, avocado, bacon, red onion, and hard-boiled egg.
2. In a small bowl, whisk together olive oil and lemon juice.
3. Pour dressing over salad and toss to combine.
4. Sprinkle with chopped chives and season with salt and pepper to taste.
5. Serve immediately.

This recipe yields 4 servings, with approximately 350 calories, 30g protein, 25g fat, and 5g net carbs per serving.

7. Chicken Caesar Salad with Romaine Lettuce

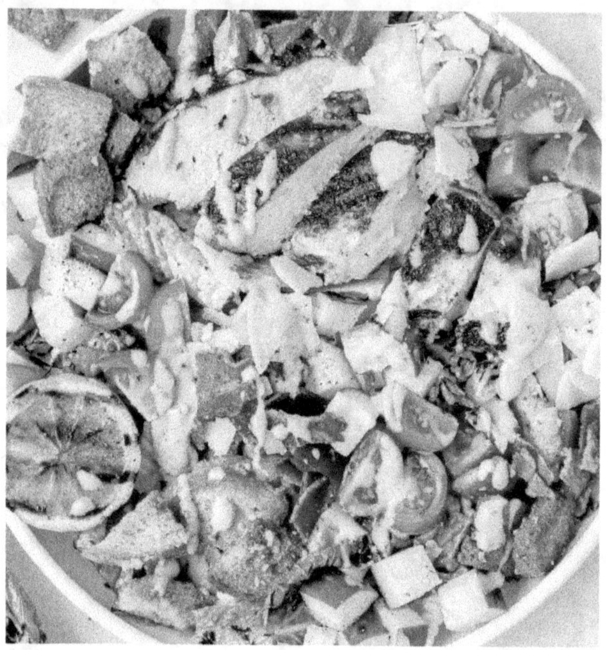

Ingredients:
- 4 cups romaine lettuce, chopped
- 1 cup cooked chicken breast, diced
- 1/2 cup homemade Caesar dressing (see below)
- 1/4 cup shaved Parmesan cheese
- 1/4 cup chopped fresh parsley

Homemade Caesar Dressing:
- 2 cloves garlic, minced
- 2 anchovy filets, minced (optional)
- 1 egg yolk
- 2 tbsp freshly squeezed lemon juice

- 1 cup olive oil
- Salt and pepper to taste

Instructions:
1. In a large bowl, combine chopped romaine lettuce, diced chicken breast, and shaved Parmesan cheese.
2. Drizzle with homemade Caesar dressing and toss to combine.
3. Sprinkle with chopped parsley and serve immediately.

This recipe yields 4 servings, with approximately 300 calories, 30g protein, 20g fat, and 5g net carbs per serving.

8. Low-Carb Chicken Quesadilla with Veggies

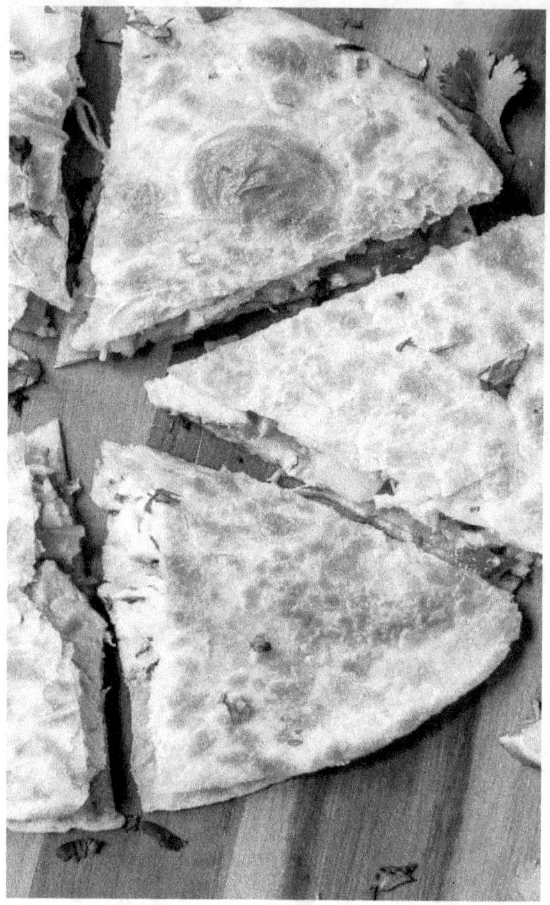

Ingredients:
- 4 boneless, skinless chicken breasts, cut into small pieces
- 1 cup mixed veggies (e.g., bell peppers, onions, mushrooms)

- 2 tbsp olive oil
- 4 low-carb tortillas (e.g., almond flour or coconut flour)
- 1 cup shredded cheese (e.g., cheddar or Monterey Jack)
- 1/4 cup chopped fresh cilantro
- Salt and pepper to taste

Instructions:
1. Heat olive oil in a large skillet over medium-high heat.
2. Add chicken and cook until browned and cooked through.
3. Add mixed veggies and cook until tender.
4. In a separate pan, warm low-carb tortillas over medium heat.
5. Place a portion of chicken and veggies on half of each tortilla, then top with shredded cheese and fold tortillas in half.
6. Cook until the cheese is melted and the tortillas are crispy.
7. Serve with chopped cilantro and enjoy!

This recipe yields 4 servings, with approximately 300 calories, 30g protein, 20g fat, and 5g net carbs per serving.

9. Baked Salmon With Green Beans And Almonds

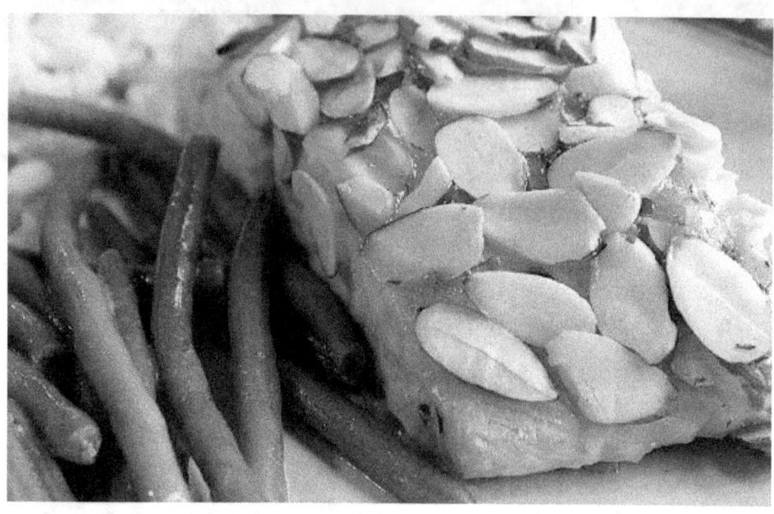

Ingredients:
- 4 salmon filets (6 oz each)
- 1 pound fresh green beans, trimmed
- 1/4 cup sliced almonds
- 2 tbsp olive oil
- 2 tbsp lemon juice
- Salt and pepper to taste

Instructions:
1. Preheat the oven to 400°F (200°C).
2. Line a baking sheet with parchment paper.
3. Place salmon filets on the baking sheet.
4. Drizzle with olive oil and lemon juice.
5. Season with salt and pepper.
6. Bake for 12-15 minutes or until cooked through.

7. Meanwhile, toss green beans with olive oil, salt, and pepper.
8. Spread on a separate baking sheet and roast for 10-12 minutes or until tender.
9. Sprinkle sliced almonds on top of green beans and return to the oven for 1-2 minutes or until toasted.
10. Serve salmon with green beans and almonds.

This recipe yields 4 servings, with approximately 350 calories, 35g protein, 20g fat, and 5g net carbs per serving.

10. Pork Chop With Roasted Veggies And Pesto

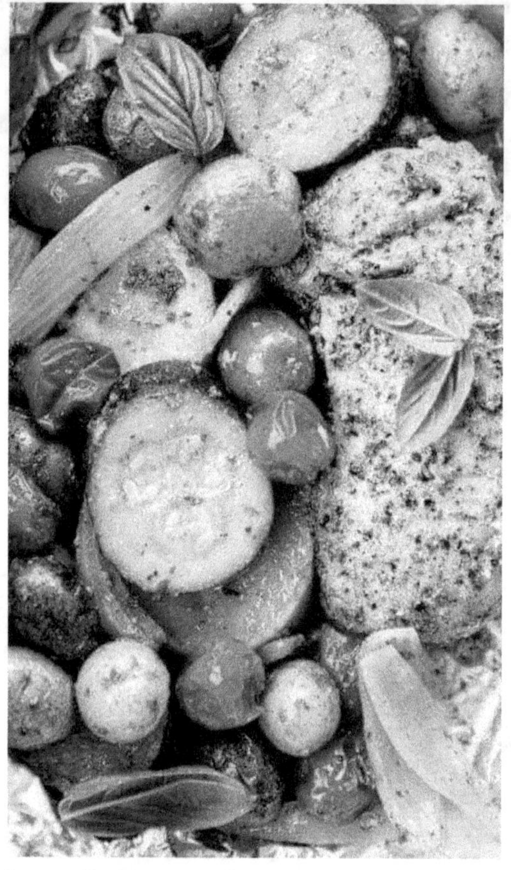

Ingredients:
- 4 pork chops (6 oz each)
- 1 cup mixed veggies (e.g., broccoli, cauliflower, Brussels sprouts)
- 1/4 cup pesto sauce
- 2 tbsp olive oil

- Salt and pepper to taste

Instructions:
1. Preheat the oven to 400°F (200°C).
2. Season pork chops with salt and pepper.
3. Heat olive oil in an oven-safe skillet over medium-high heat.
4. Sear pork chops for 2-3 minutes per side, then transfer to the oven.
5. Roast for 15-20 minutes or until cooked through.
6. Toss mixed veggies with olive oil, salt, and pepper.
7. Spread on a separate baking sheet and roast for 15-20 minutes or until tender.
8. Serve pork chops with roasted veggies and pesto sauce.

This recipe yields 4 servings, with approximately 350 calories, 35g protein, 20g fat, and 5g net carbs per serving.

11. Low-Carb Chicken And Bacon Salad

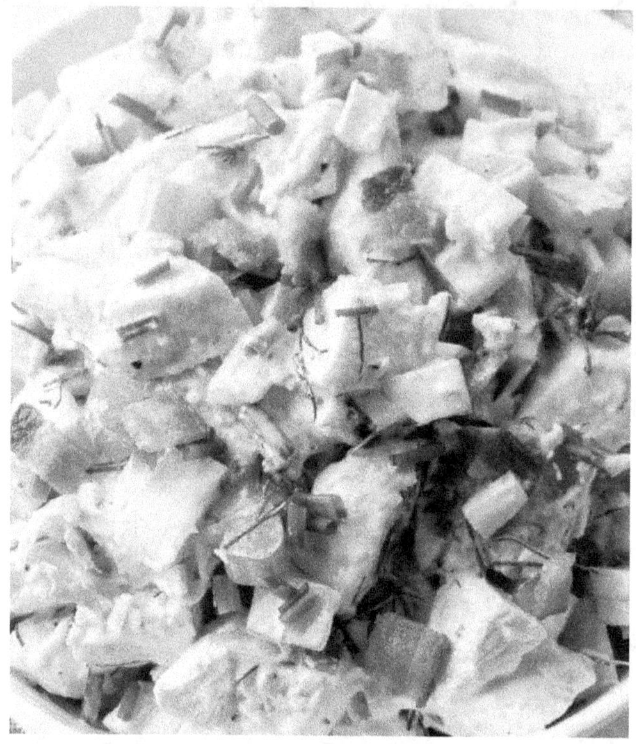

Ingredients:
- 1 pound cooked chicken breast, diced
- 6 slices of bacon, cooked and crumbled
- 1 cup mixed greens
- 1 cup cherry tomatoes, halved
- 1/4 cup sliced red onion
- 2 tbsp olive oil
- 1 tbsp lemon juice
- Salt and pepper to taste

Instructions:
1. In a large bowl, combine chicken breast, bacon, mixed greens, cherry tomatoes, and red onion.
2. In a small bowl, whisk together olive oil and lemon juice.
3. Pour dressing over salad and toss to combine.
4. Season with salt and pepper to taste.
5. Serve immediately.

This recipe yields 4 servings, with approximately 300 calories, 30g protein, 20g fat, and 5g net carbs per serving.

12. Grilled Chicken Breast With Roasted Veggies

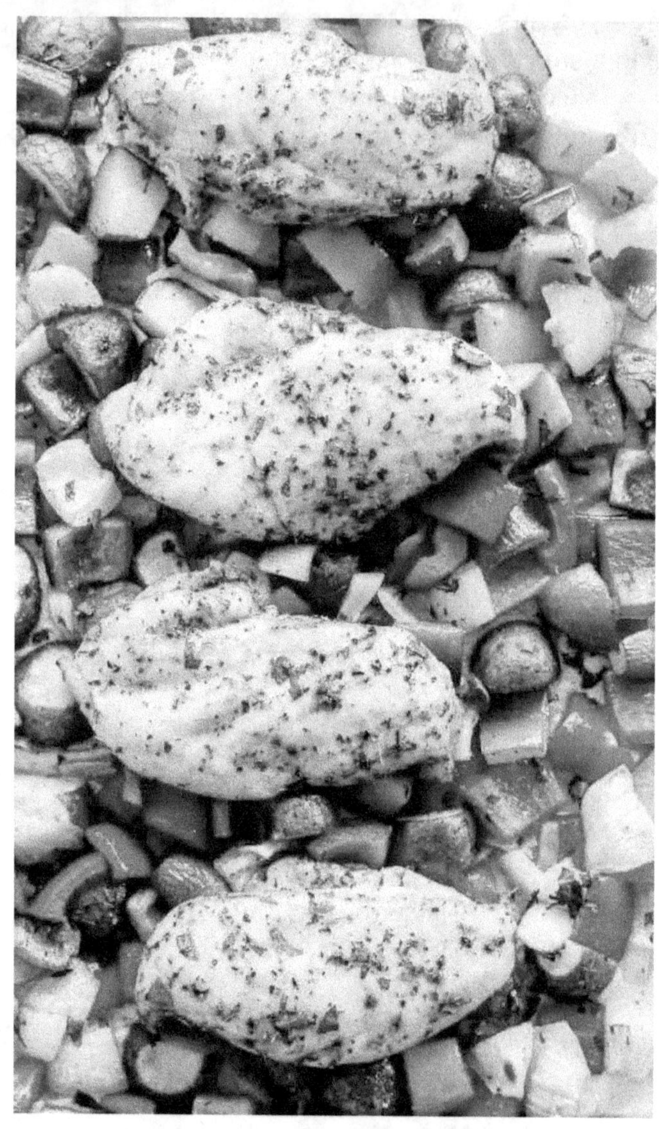

Ingredients:
- 4 boneless, skinless chicken breasts
- 2 cups mixed veggies (e.g., broccoli, cauliflower, Brussels sprouts)
- 2 tbsp olive oil
- 1 tsp salt
- 1 tsp pepper
- 1 tsp garlic powder (optional)

Instructions:
1. Preheat the grill to medium-high heat.
2. Season chicken breasts with salt, pepper, and garlic powder (if using).
3. Grill chicken for 5-6 minutes per side or until cooked through.
4. Toss veggies with olive oil, salt, and pepper.
5. Spread on a baking sheet and roast in the oven at 400°F (200°C) for 15-20 minutes or until tender.
6. Serve grilled chicken with roasted veggies.

This recipe yields 4 servings, with approximately 250 calories, 35g protein, 10g fat, and 5g net carbs per serving.

13. Spinach And Feta Stuffed Chicken Breast

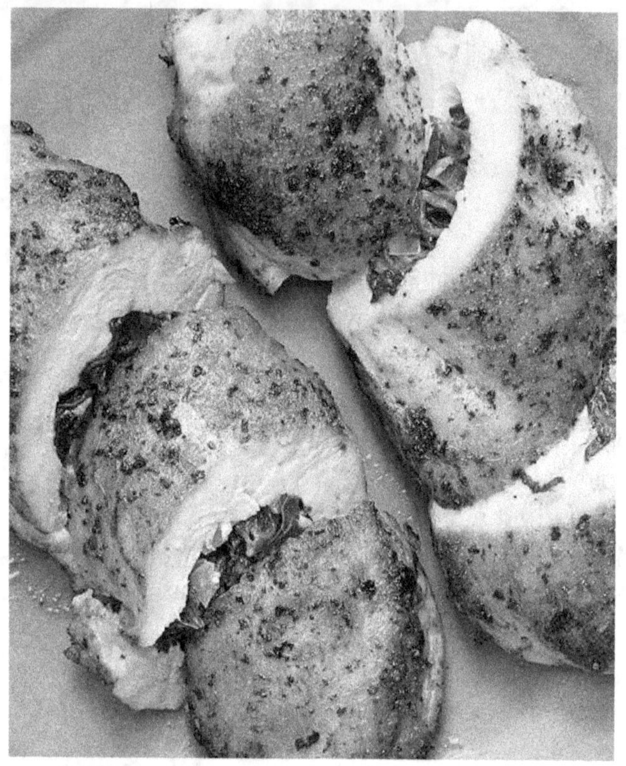

Ingredients:
- 4 boneless, skinless chicken breasts
- 1 package frozen chopped spinach, thawed and drained
- 1/2 cup crumbled feta cheese
- 1/4 cup chopped fresh parsley
- 2 cloves garlic, minced
- 1/2 tsp salt
- 1/4 tsp black pepper

- 2 tbsp olive oil

Instructions:
1. Preheat the oven to 375°F (190°C).
2. In a bowl, mix spinach, feta cheese, parsley, garlic, salt, and pepper.
3. Lay chicken breasts flat and make a horizontal incision to create a pocket.
4. Stuff each breast with the spinach-feta mixture.
5. Drizzle with olive oil and bake for 30-35 minutes or until cooked through.

This recipe yields 4 servings, with approximately 350 calories, 35g protein, 20g fat, and 5g net carbs per serving.

14. Turkey And Cheese Roll-Ups With Lettuce

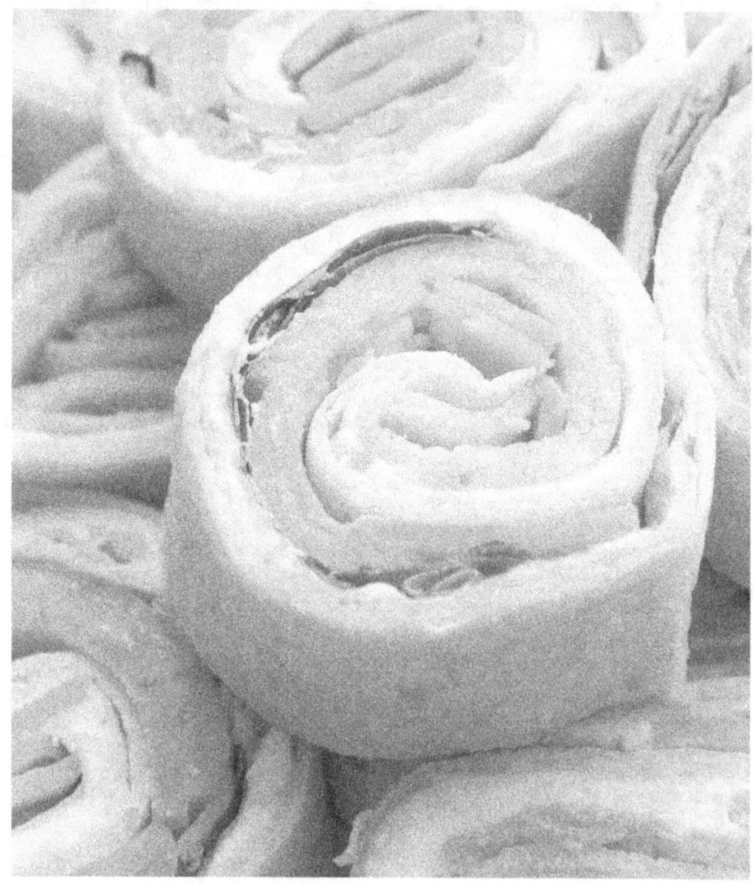

Ingredients:
- 4 slices deli turkey breast
- 4 slices cheese (e.g., cheddar, Swiss, or provolone)
- 4 large lettuce leaves
- 1/4 cup chopped fresh parsley

- 1/4 cup sliced red bell pepper
- 2 tbsp mayonnaise or low-carb ranch dressing

Instructions:
1. Lay a slice of turkey flat and add a slice of cheese, some parsley, and bell pepper.
2. Roll up tightly and repeat with remaining ingredients.
3. Wrap each roll-up with a lettuce leaf and secure with a toothpick if needed.
4. Serve with mayonnaise or ranch dressing for dipping.

This recipe yields 4 servings, with approximately 250 calories, 25g protein, 15g fat, and 5g net carbs per serving.

15. Chicken And Avocado Wrap With Lettuce And Tomato

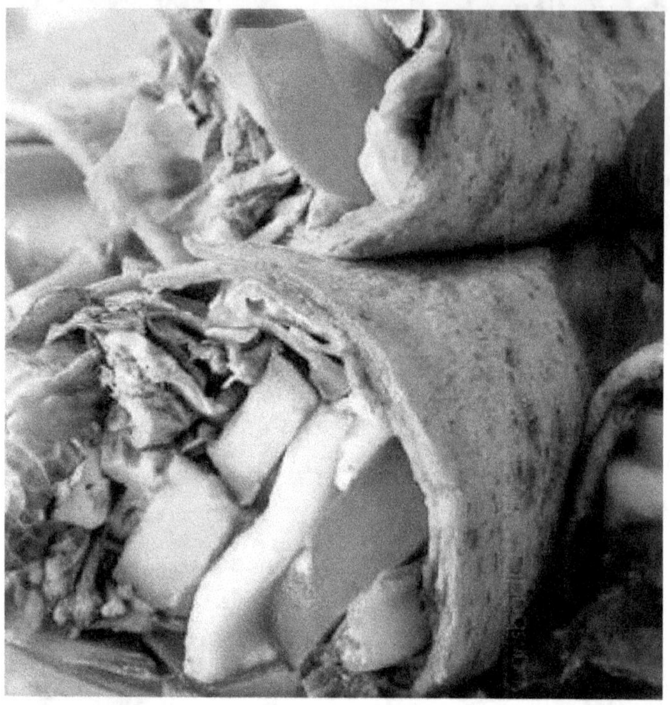

Ingredients:

- 1 pound cooked chicken breast, shredded
- 1 ripe avocado, sliced
- 4 large lettuce leaves
- 2 medium tomatoes, sliced
- 1/4 cup chopped fresh cilantro
- 2 tbsp lime juice
- Salt and pepper to taste

Instructions:

1. Lay a lettuce leaf flat and add shredded chicken,
sliced avocado, tomato, and cilantro.
2. Drizzle with lime juice and season with salt and
pepper.
3. Fold the lettuce leaf to enclose the filling.
4. Repeat with remaining ingredients.

This recipe yields 4 servings, with approximately
300 calories, 30g protein, 20g fat, and 5g net carbs
per serving.

Satisfying Dinner Recipes

1. Grilled Steak With Roasted Garlic Mashed Cauliflower

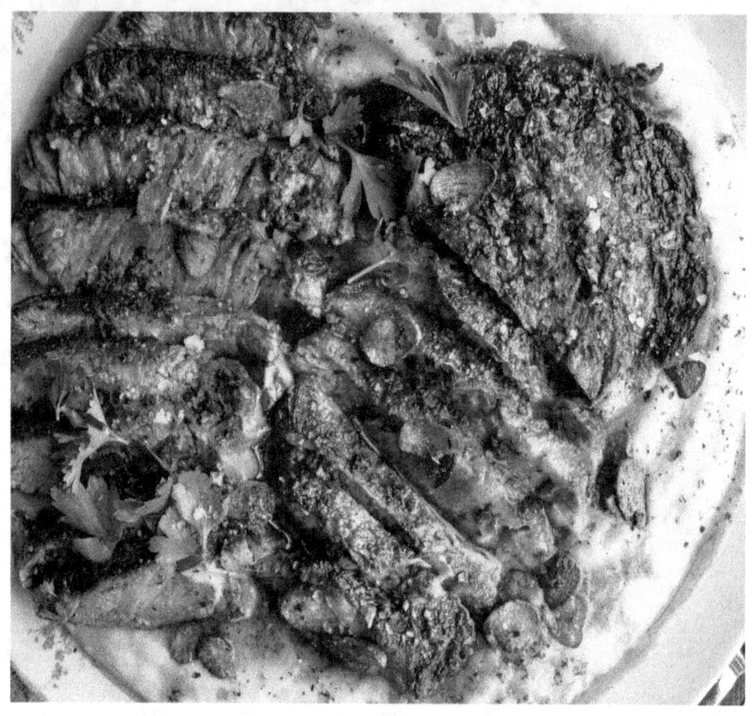

Ingredients:
- 1.5 lbs steak (Ribeye or Sirloin)
- 4-5 cloves garlic, peeled and chopped
- 1 head cauliflower, broken into florets
- 2 tbsp olive oil
- 1/2 cup grated cheddar cheese (optional)

- Salt and pepper to taste

Instructions:
1. Preheat the grill to medium-high heat.
2. Season steak with salt and pepper. Grill for 5-7 minutes per side or until cooked to desired doneness.
3. Toss cauliflower with olive oil, salt, and pepper. Roast in the oven at 425°F (220°C) for 20-25 minutes or until tender.
4. Mash roasted cauliflower with butter, garlic, and cheese (if using).
5. Serve grilled steak with roasted garlic mashed cauliflower.

This recipe yields 4 servings, with approximately 350 calories, 35g protein, 20g fat, and 5g net carbs per serving.

2. Baked Chicken Breast With Spinach, Feta, And Sun-Dried Tomatoes

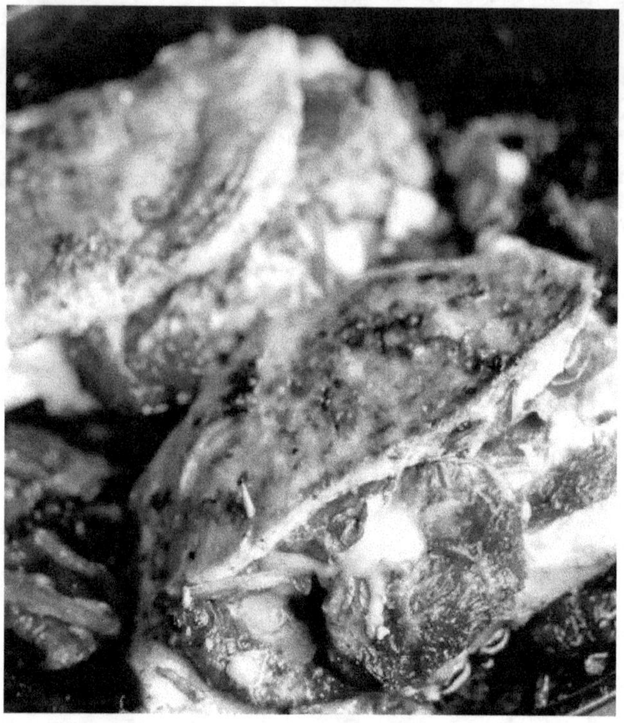

Ingredients:
- 4 boneless, skinless chicken breasts
- 1 package frozen chopped spinach, thawed and drained
- 1/2 cup crumbled feta cheese
- 1/4 cup chopped sun-dried tomatoes
- 2 cloves garlic, minced
- 1/2 tsp salt

- 1/4 tsp black pepper
- 2 tbsp olive oil

Instructions:
1. Preheat the oven to 375°F (190°C).
2. In a bowl, mix spinach, feta cheese, sun-dried tomatoes, garlic, salt, and pepper.
3. Lay chicken breasts flat and make a horizontal incision to create a pocket.
4. Stuff each breast with the spinach-feta mixture.
5. Drizzle with olive oil and bake for 30-35 minutes or until cooked through.

This recipe yields 4 servings, with approximately 300 calories, 35g protein, 15g fat, and 5g net carbs per serving.

3. Pork Tenderloin With Apple Cider Jus And Roasted Vegetables

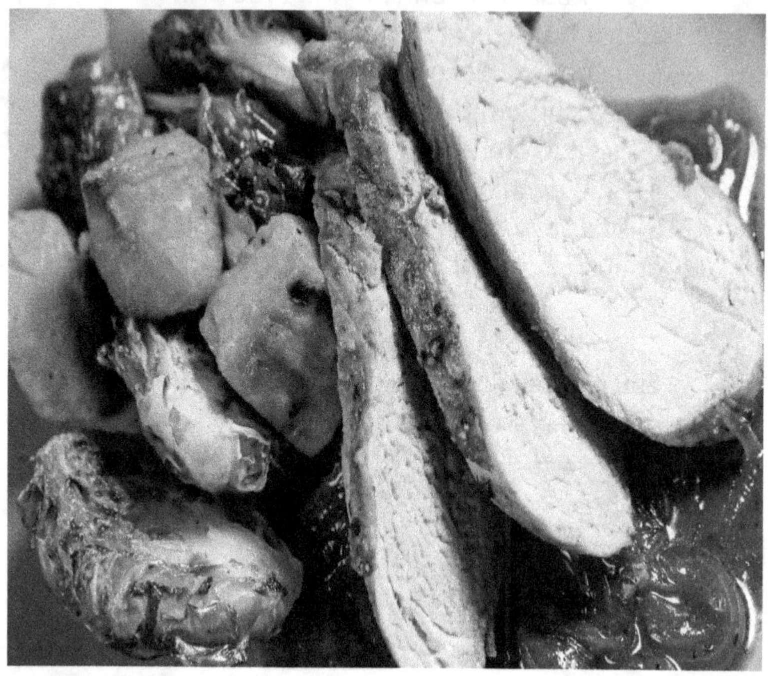

Ingredients:

- 1 (1-1.5 pound) pork tenderloin
- 1/4 cup apple cider jus (or apple cider reduction)
- 2 tbsp olive oil
- 1 large onion, peeled and chopped
- 2 cloves garlic, minced
- 2 carrots, peeled and chopped
- 2 Brussels sprouts, trimmed and halved
- Salt and pepper to taste

Instructions:
1. Preheat the oven to 400°F (200°C).
2. Season pork tenderloin with salt and pepper.
3. In a large skillet, heat olive oil over medium-high heat. Sear pork tenderloin until browned on all sides, about 5 minutes. Transfer to a baking sheet and roast in the oven for 15-20 minutes or until cooked through.
4. In the same skillet, add chopped onion and cook until caramelized, about 5 minutes. Add garlic, carrots, and Brussels sprouts, and cook for an additional 5 minutes.
5. Serve pork tenderloin with roasted vegetables and drizzle with apple cider jus.

This recipe yields 4 servings, with approximately 250 calories, 30g protein, 10g fat, and 5g net carbs per serving.

4. Low-Carb Beef And Mushroom Gravy Over Cauliflower Mash

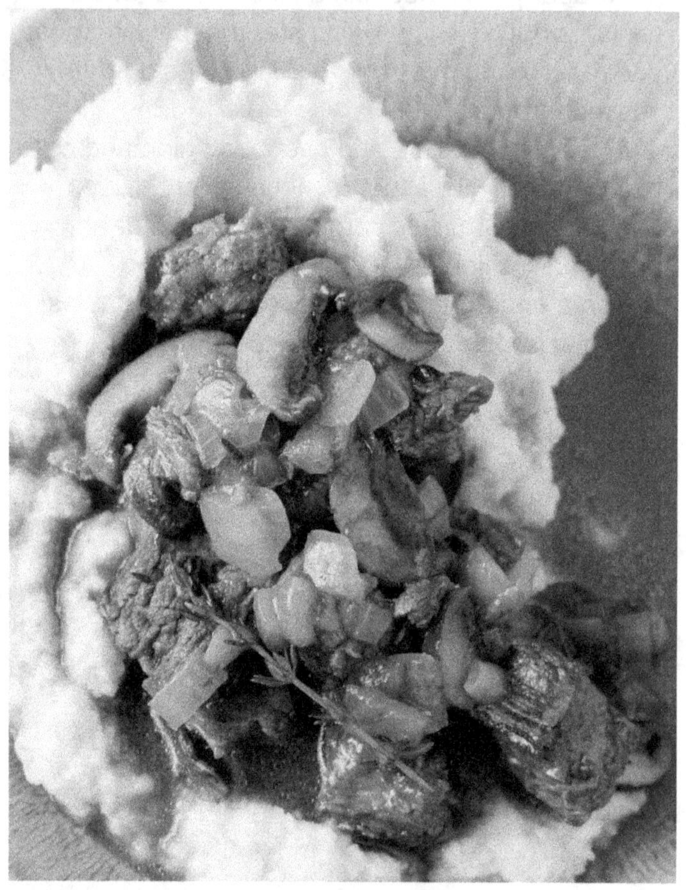

Ingredients:
- 1 lb beef strips (sirloin or ribeye)
- 1 cup mixed mushrooms (button, cremini, shiitake)

- 2 cloves garlic, minced
- 1 cup beef broth
- 1 tbsp tomato paste
- 2 tbsp butter
- 1 head cauliflower, broken into florets
- Salt and pepper to taste

Instructions:
1. Cook beef and mushrooms in butter until browned.
2. Add garlic, beef broth, and tomato paste. Simmer for 5-7 minutes.
3. Toss cauliflower with butter, salt, and pepper. Roast in the oven at 425°F (220°C) for 20-25 minutes or until tender.
4. Mash roasted cauliflower with butter and cream (optional).
5. Serve beef and mushroom gravy over cauliflower mash.

This recipe yields 4 servings, with approximately 350 calories, 25g protein, 20g fat, and 5g net carbs per serving.

5. Grilled Salmon With Avocado And Bacon Salad

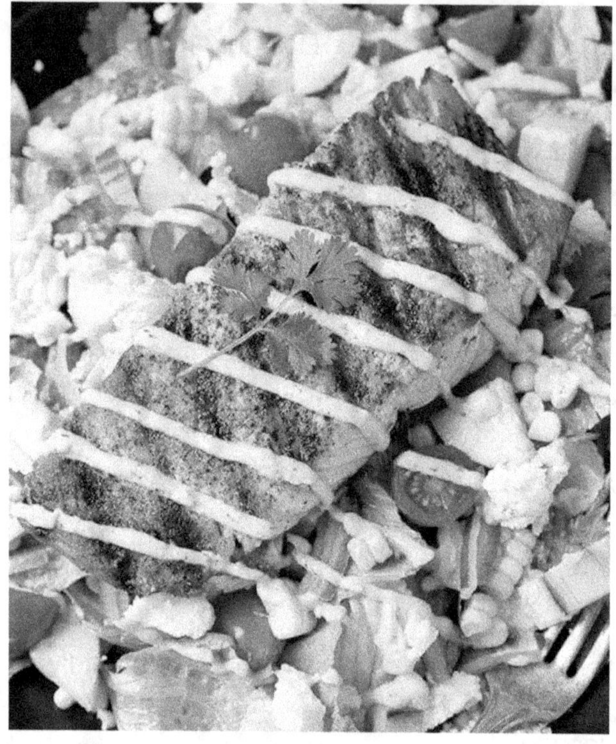

Ingredients:
- 4 salmon filets (6 oz each)
- 2 ripe avocados, diced
- 6 slices of bacon, cooked and crumbled
- 1/4 cup chopped fresh dill
- 2 tbsp freshly squeezed lemon juice
- Salt and pepper to taste

Instructions:

1. Grill salmon filets until cooked through.
2. In a large bowl, combine diced avocado,
crumbled bacon, chopped dill, and lemon juice.
3. Serve grilled salmon on top of the
avocado-bacon salad.

This recipe yields 4 servings, with approximately
350 calories, 30g protein, 25g fat, and 5g net carbs
per serving.

6. Chicken And Vegetable Skewers With Peanut Sauce

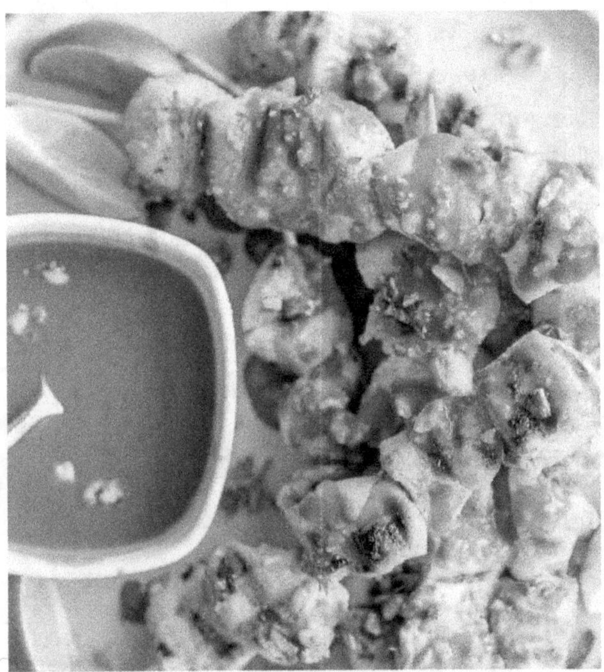

Ingredients:

- 1 lb boneless, skinless chicken breast, cut into bite-sized pieces
- 1 red bell pepper, cut into large pieces
- 1 yellow bell pepper, cut into large pieces
- 1 onion, cut into large pieces
- 2 cloves garlic, minced
- 1/4 cup peanut butter
- 1/4 cup coconut milk
- 2 tbsp soy sauce
- 2 tbsp honey
- 1 tsp grated ginger
- Salt and pepper to taste

Instructions:
1. Preheat the grill to medium-high heat.
2. Thread chicken, bell peppers, onion, and garlic onto skewers.
3. Grill for 10-12 minutes or until chicken is cooked through.
4. In a bowl, whisk together peanut butter, coconut milk, soy sauce, honey, and ginger.
5. Serve peanut sauce over grilled skewers.

This recipe yields 4 servings, with approximately 300 calories, 25g protein, 15g fat, and 5g net carbs per serving.

7. Grilled Steak Fajitas With Bell Peppers And Onions

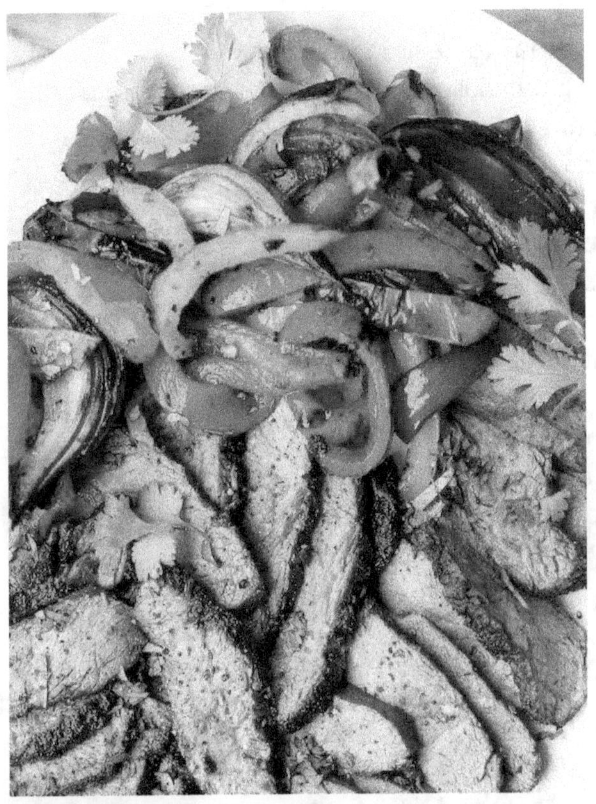

Ingredients:
- 1 lb steak (flank steak or skirt steak)
- 2 bell peppers (any color), sliced
- 1 large onion, sliced
- 2 cloves garlic, minced
- 1 tsp ground cumin
- 1 tsp chili powder
- 1/4 tsp cayenne pepper (optional)

- Salt and pepper to taste
- 4 low-carb tortillas (optional)

Instructions:
1. Grill steak to desired doneness.
2. In a large skillet, sauté bell peppers, onion, and garlic until tender.
3. Add cumin, chili powder, and cayenne pepper (if using) to the skillet and stir for 1 minute.
4. Slice grilled steak into thin strips and add to the skillet.
5. Serve with low-carb tortillas (if using) and your favorite toppings.

This recipe yields 4 servings, with approximately 300 calories, 25g protein, 15g fat, and 5g net carbs per serving (without tortillas).

8. Baked Cod With Lemon, Herbs And Zucchini Noodles

Ingredients:
- 4 cod filets (6 oz each)
- 2 lemons, juiced
- 1/4 cup olive oil
- 4 tbsp chopped fresh parsley
- 2 tbsp chopped fresh dill
- 2 cloves garlic, minced
- 1 medium zucchini, spiralized
- Salt and pepper to taste

Instructions:
1. Preheat the oven to 400°F (200°C).
2. Line a baking sheet with parchment paper.
3. Place cod filets on the baking sheet.
4. Drizzle with olive oil, lemon juice, parsley, dill, and garlic.
5. Bake for 12-15 minutes or until cod is cooked through.
6. Serve with zucchini noodles (zoodles) and your favorite sides.

This recipe yields 4 servings, with approximately 200 calories, 25g protein, 10g fat, and 5g net carbs per serving.

9. Low-Carb Meatloaf With Ketchup Glaze And Roasted Broccoli

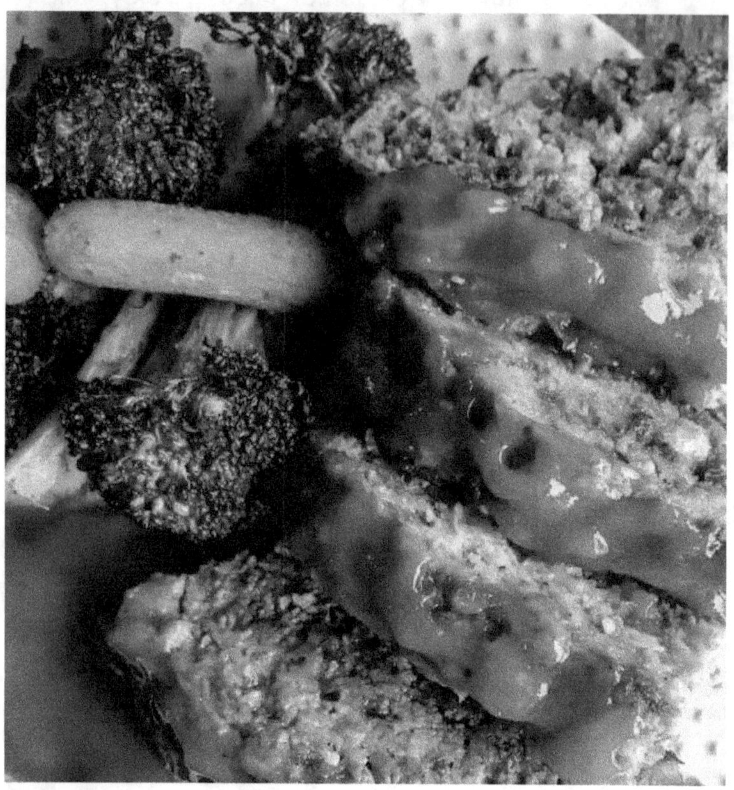

Ingredients:
- 1 lb ground meat (beef, pork, or a combination)
- 1/2 cup almond flour
- 1/4 cup grated cheddar cheese
- 1 egg
- 1/4 cup ketchup
- 2 tbsp brown sugar

- 1 tsp smoked paprika
- Salt and pepper to taste
- 4 cups broccoli florets

Instructions:
1. Preheat the oven to 375°F (190°C).
2. In a large bowl, combine ground meat, almond flour, cheese, egg, ketchup, brown sugar, smoked paprika, salt, and pepper. Mix well.
3. Form into a loaf shape and place on a baking sheet.
4. Roast in the oven for 40-45 minutes or until cooked through.
5. While the meatloaf is cooking, toss broccoli with olive oil, salt, and pepper. Roast in the oven for 15-20 minutes or until tender.
6. During the last 10 minutes of cooking, brush the meatloaf with ketchup glaze (made by mixing ketchup and brown sugar).

This recipe yields 4 servings, with approximately 350 calories, 25g protein, 20g fat, and 5g net carbs per serving.

10. Grilled Chicken Breast With Pesto And Zucchini Noodles

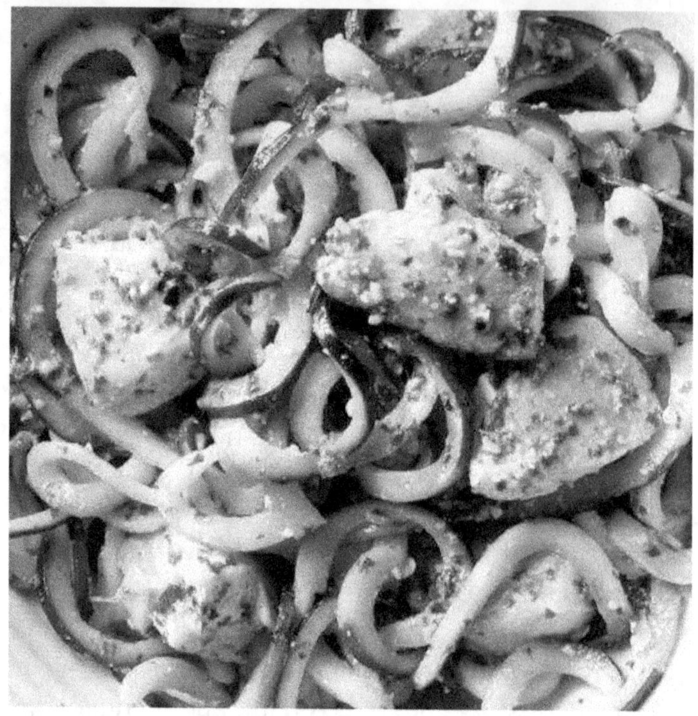

Ingredients:

- 4 boneless, skinless chicken breasts
- 1/2 cup freshly made pesto
- 2 medium zucchinis, spiralized
- 2 cloves garlic, minced
- 1/4 cup grated Parmesan cheese
- Salt and pepper to taste

Instructions:

1. Preheat the grill to medium-high heat.

2. Grill chicken breasts for 5-7 minutes per side or until cooked through.
3. Meanwhile, sauté zucchini noodles and garlic in a skillet with a little olive oil until tender.
4. Stir in pesto and cook for an additional minute.
5. Serve grilled chicken breasts with pesto zucchini noodles and top with Parmesan cheese.

This recipe yields 4 servings, with approximately 250 calories, 30g protein, 15g fat, and 5g net carbs per serving.

11. Low-Carb Beef And Vegetable Stir-Fry With Cauliflower Rice

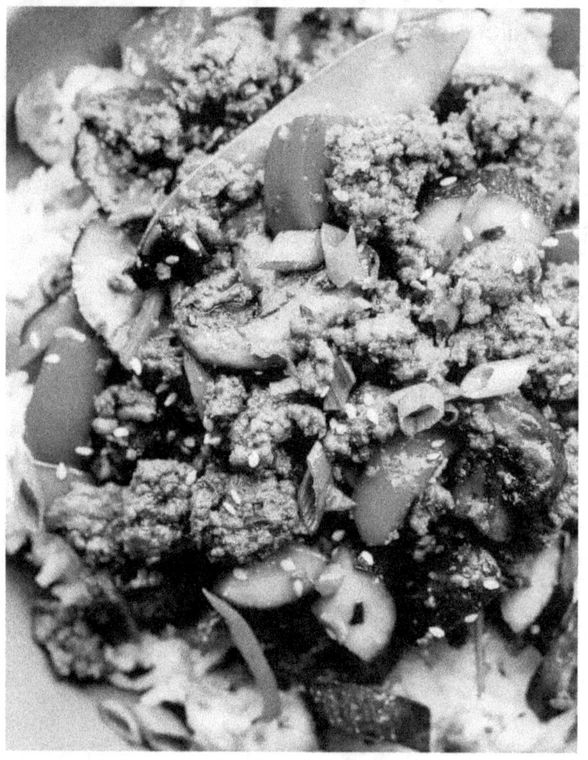

Ingredients:
- 1 lb beef strips (sirloin or ribeye)
- 2 cups mixed vegetables (bell peppers, carrots, broccoli, onions)
- 2 cloves garlic, minced
- 1 cup cauliflower rice
- 2 tbsp coconut oil

- 1 tsp soy sauce
- 1 tsp oyster sauce (optional)
- Salt and pepper to taste

Instructions:
1. Cook beef and vegetables in coconut oil until beef is browned and veggies are tender.
2. Add garlic, cauliflower rice, soy sauce, and oyster sauce (if using). Stir-fry for 2-3 minutes.
3. Serve hot and enjoy!

This recipe yields 4 servings, with approximately 300 calories, 25g protein, 15g fat, and 5g net carbs per serving.

12. Baked Salmon With Lemon, Herbs And Green Beans

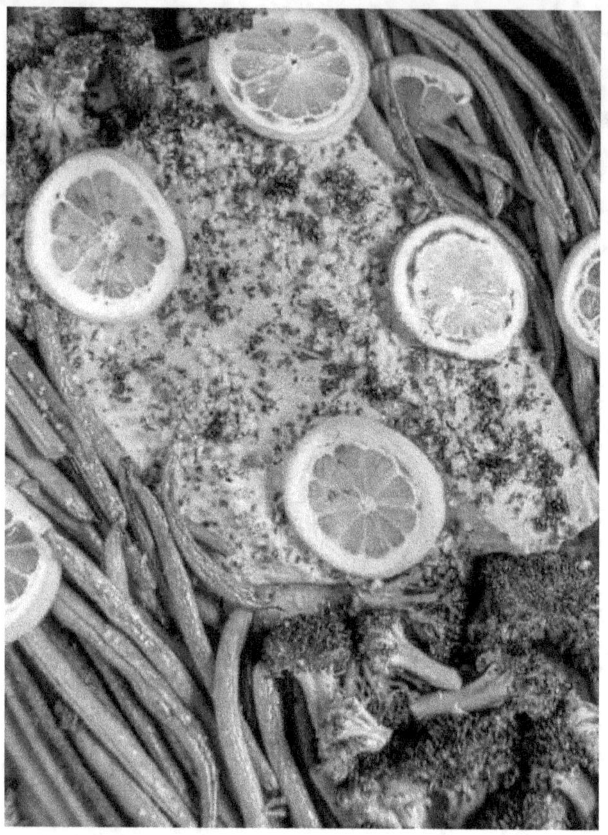

Ingredients:

- 4 salmon filets (6 oz each)
- 2 lemons, juiced
- 1/4 cup olive oil
- 4 tbsp chopped fresh parsley
- 2 tbsp chopped fresh dill
- 2 cloves garlic, minced

- 1 lb fresh green beans, trimmed
- Salt and pepper to taste

Instructions:
1. Preheat the oven to 400°F (200°C).
2. Line a baking sheet with parchment paper.
3. Place salmon filets on the baking sheet.
4. Drizzle with olive oil, lemon juice, parsley, dill, and garlic.
5. Roast in the oven for 12-15 minutes or until salmon is cooked through.
6. Toss green beans with olive oil, salt, and pepper. Roast in the oven for 5-7 minutes or until tender.

This recipe yields 4 servings, with approximately 200 calories, 25g protein, 10g fat, and 5g net carbs per serving.

13. Low-Carb Chicken And Mushroom Creamy Sauce Over Zucchini Noodles

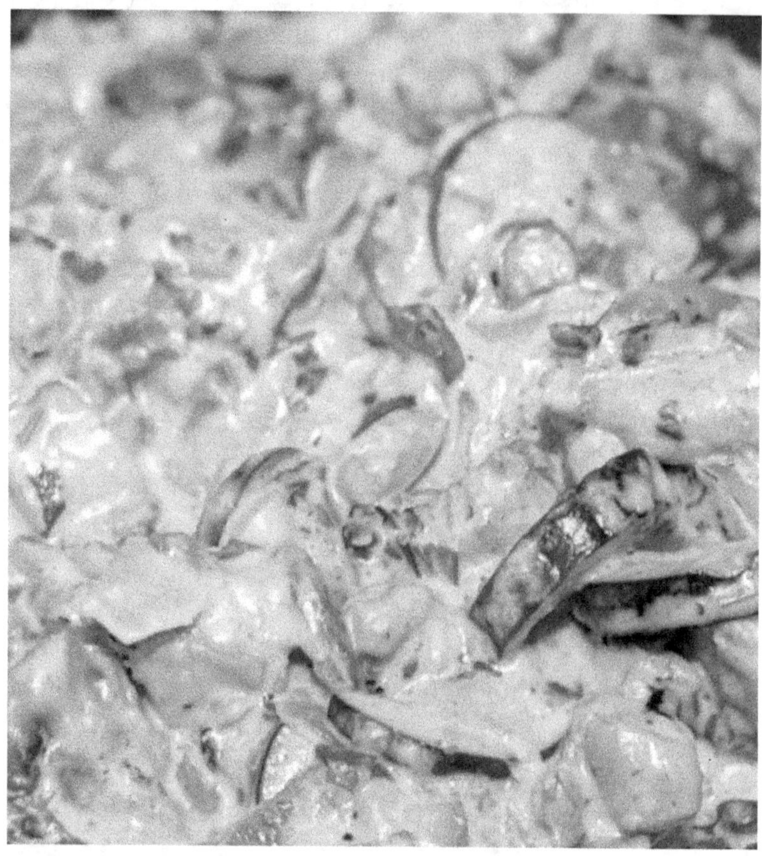

Ingredients:
- 1 lb boneless, skinless chicken breast
- 2 cups mixed mushrooms (button, cremini, shiitake)
- 2 cloves garlic, minced

- 1 cup heavy cream
- 1/2 cup grated Parmesan cheese
- 1 tsp dried thyme
- Salt and pepper to taste
- 4 medium zucchinis, spiralized

Instructions:
1. Cook chicken and mushrooms in a skillet until chicken is cooked through and mushrooms are tender.
2. Add garlic, heavy cream, Parmesan cheese, and thyme. Stir until sauce thickens.
3. Serve over zucchini noodles (zoodles) and enjoy.

This recipe yields 4 servings, with approximately 250 calories, 25g protein, 15g fat, and 5g net carbs per serving.

14. Grilled Steak With Roasted Brussels Sprouts And Sweet Potato

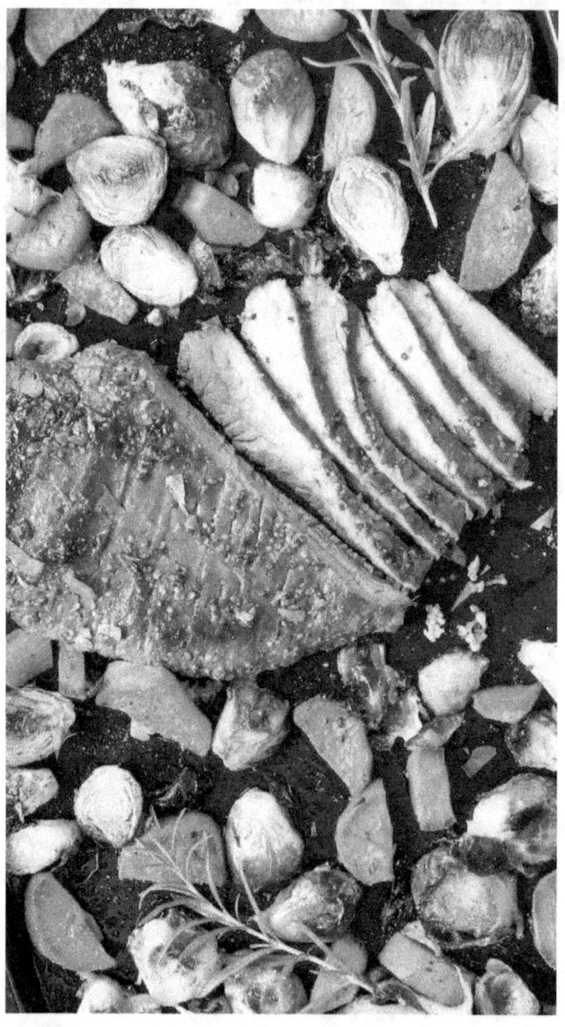

Ingredients:

- 1.5 lbs steak (ribeye or strip loin)
- 1 large sweet potato, peeled and cubed
- 1 pound Brussels sprouts, trimmed and halved
- 2 tbsp olive oil
- Salt and pepper to taste
- 1 tsp garlic powder (optional)

Instructions:
1. Preheat the grill to medium-high heat. Grill steak for 5-7 minutes per side or until cooked to desired doneness.
2. Toss sweet potato and Brussels sprouts with olive oil, salt, pepper, and garlic powder (if using). Spread on a baking sheet and roast in the oven at 425°F (220°C) for 20-25 minutes or until tender.
3. Serve grilled steak with roasted sweet potato and Brussels sprouts.

This recipe yields 4 servings, with approximately 350 calories, 30g protein, 20g fat, and 10g net carbs per serving.

15. Low-Carb Chicken And Vegetable Kabobs With Pesto Sauce

Ingredients:
- 1 lb boneless, skinless chicken breast, cut into bite-sized pieces
- 1 cup mixed vegetables (bell peppers, onions, mushrooms, cherry tomatoes)

- 1/4 cup freshly made pesto sauce
- 2 tbsp olive oil
- Salt and pepper to taste

Instructions:
1. Preheat the grill to medium-high heat. Thread chicken and vegetables onto skewers.
2. Brush with olive oil and season with salt and pepper. Grill for 10-12 minutes or until chicken is cooked through.
3. Serve with pesto sauce for dipping.

This recipe yields 4 servings, with approximately 200 calories, 25g protein, 10g fat, and 5g net carbs per serving.

Chapter Three

Appetizers And Snacks

1. Breakfast Scramble With Spinach, Mushrooms And Goat Cheese

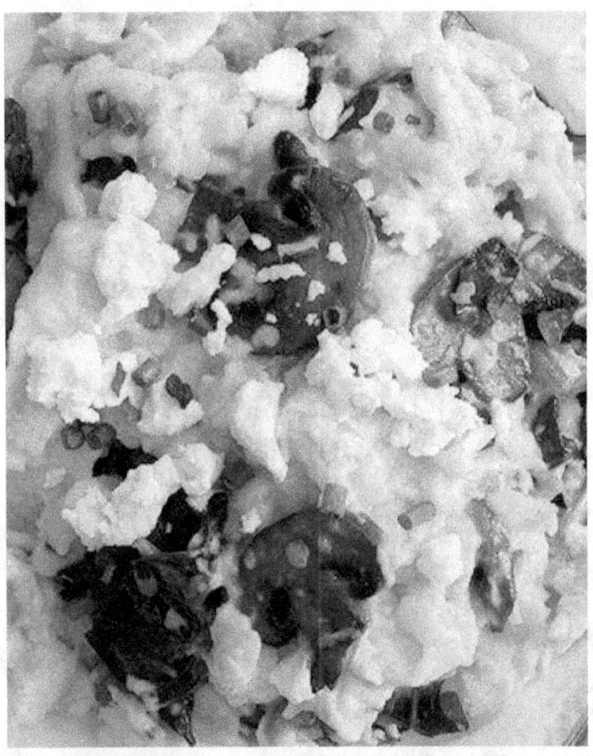

Ingredients:

- 4 eggs
- 1 cup fresh spinach leaves
- 1 cup sliced mushrooms
- 1/4 cup crumbled goat cheese
- 1/2 tsp salt
- 1/4 tsp black pepper
- 1 tbsp butter

Instructions:
1. In a bowl, whisk eggs and set aside.
2. In a skillet, sauté spinach, mushrooms, and butter until tender.
3. Pour in eggs and cook until scrambled.
4. Stir in goat cheese, salt, and pepper.
5. Serve hot and enjoy!

This recipe yields 4 servings, with approximately 150 calories, 12g protein, 10g fat, and 2g net carbs per serving.

2. Low-Carb Protein Smoothie With Banana, Almond Milk And Chia Seeds

Ingredients:
- 1 scoop vanilla protein powder
- 1/2 banana
- 1/2 cup almond milk
- 1 tablespoon chia seeds
- 1/2 teaspoon vanilla extract
- Ice cubes (optional)

Instructions:
1. In a blender, combine protein powder, banana, almond milk, chia seeds, and vanilla extract.
2. Blend until smooth and creamy.
3. Add ice cubes if you want a thicker consistency.
4. Blend again until ice is crushed and the smoothie is the desired consistency.
5. Pour into a glass and serve immediately.

This recipe yields 1 serving, with approximately 200 calories, 20g protein, 10g fat, and 5g net carbs.

3. Low-Carb Cauliflower Fried Rice with Shrimp and Vegetables

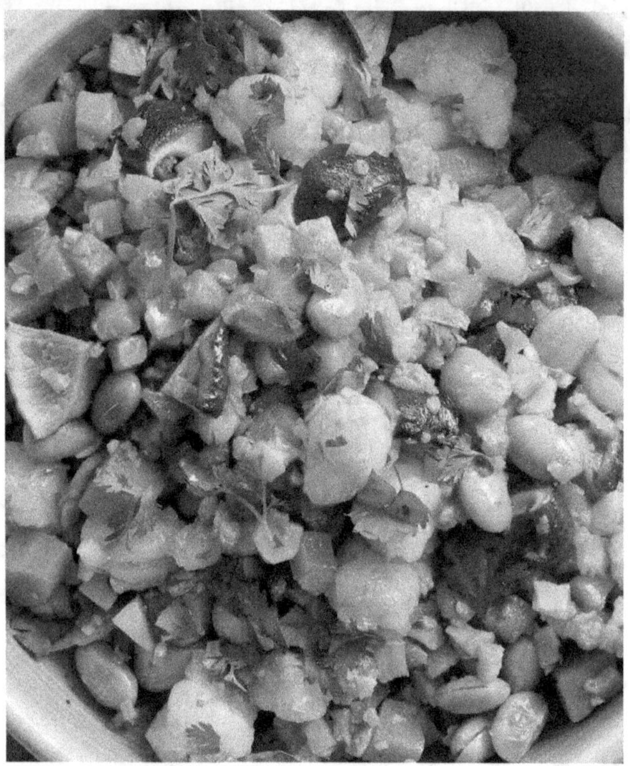

Ingredients:
- 1 head cauliflower
- 1 cup cooked shrimp
- 1 cup mixed vegetables (e.g., peas, carrots, green onions)
- 2 tablespoons coconut oil
- 2 cloves garlic, minced
- 1 teaspoon soy sauce
- Salt and pepper to taste

Instructions:
1. Pulse cauliflower in a food processor until it resembles rice.
2. Heat coconut oil in a large skillet or wok over medium-high heat.
3. Add garlic, mixed vegetables, and cooked shrimp. Cook until vegetables are tender.
4. Add cauliflower "rice" and cook until heated through.
5. Stir in soy sauce and season with salt and pepper to taste.
6. Serve hot and enjoy!

This recipe yields 4 servings, with approximately 150 calories, 15g protein, 10g fat, and 5g net carbs per serving.

4. Baked Salmon And Green Beans

Ingredients:
- 4 salmon filets (6 oz each)
- 1/4 cup olive oil
- 4 tbsp chopped fresh parsley
- 2 tbsp chopped fresh dill
- 2 cloves garlic, minced
- 1 lb fresh green beans, trimmed
- Salt and pepper to taste

Instructions:

1. Preheat the oven to 400°F (200°C).
2. Line a baking sheet with parchment paper.
3. Place salmon filets on the baking sheet.
4. Drizzle with olive oil, parsley, dill, and garlic.
5. Roast in the oven for 12-15 minutes or until salmon is cooked through.
6. Toss green beans with olive oil, salt, and pepper. Roast in the oven for 5-7 minutes or until tender.

This recipe yields 4 servings, with approximately 200 calories, 25g protein, 10g fat, and 5g net carbs per serving.

5. Low-Carb Chicken And Vegetable Stir-Fry

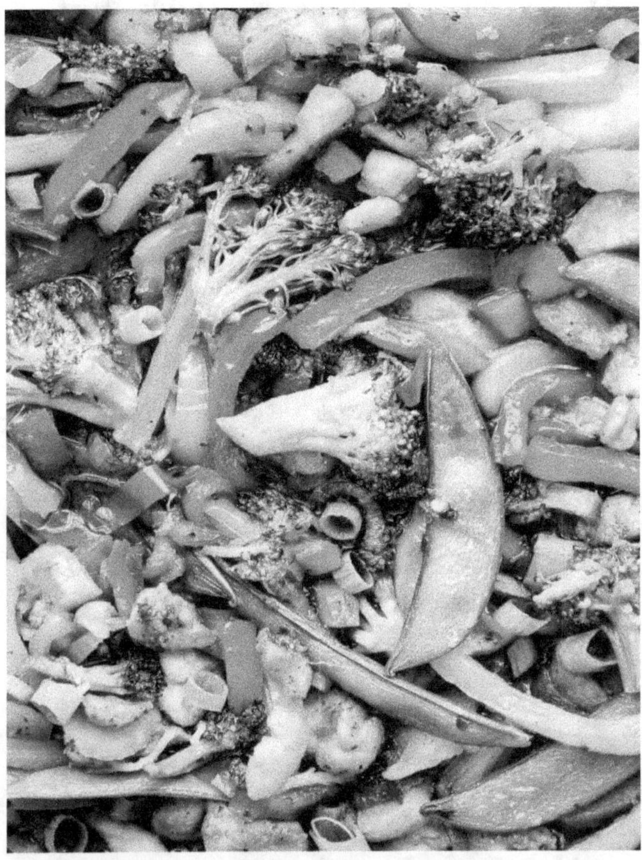

Ingredients:
- 1 lb boneless, skinless chicken breast
- 1 cup mixed vegetables (bell peppers, carrots, broccoli, onions)
- 2 cloves garlic, minced
- 1 tablespoon coconut oil

- Salt and pepper to taste

Instructions:
1. Heat coconut oil in a large skillet or wok over medium-high heat.
2. Add chicken and cook until browned and cooked through.
3. Add mixed vegetables and garlic. Cook until vegetables are tender.
4. Serve hot and enjoy!

This recipe yields 4 servings, with approximately 150 calories, 20g protein, 10g fat, and 5g net carbs per serving.

6. Prosciutto And Melon Platter

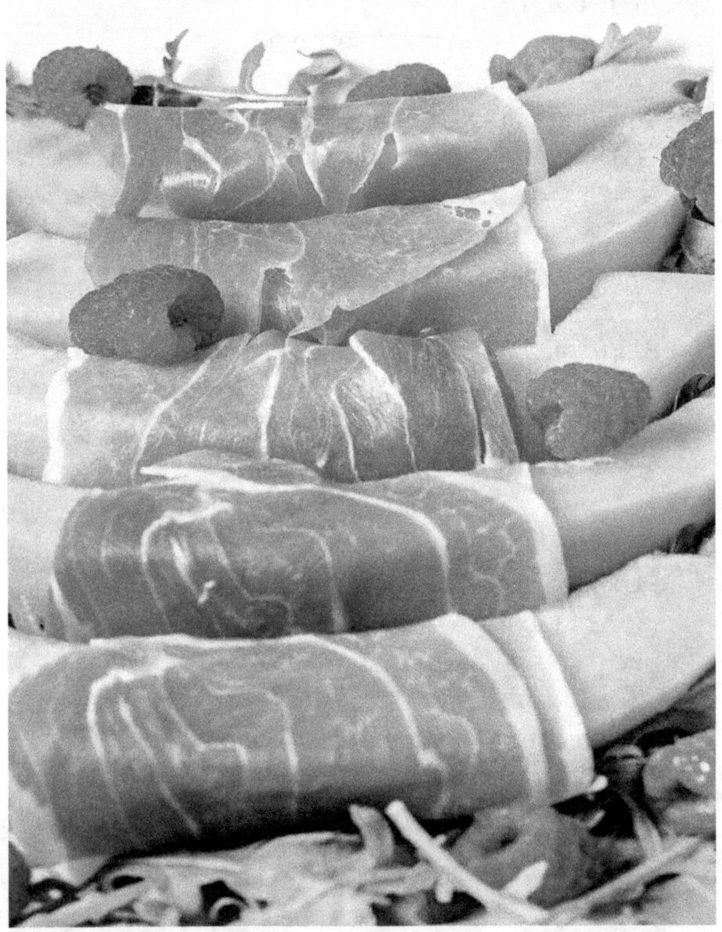

Ingredients:
- 1 ripe melon (such as cantaloupe or honeydew)
- 6-8 slices of prosciutto
- 8 oz fresh Mozzarella cheese
- 1 cup cherry tomatoes, halved

- 1/4 cup fresh basil leaves

Instructions:
1. Cut the melon into 1-inch thick slices.
2. Wrap each melon slice with a slice of prosciutto, securing with a toothpick if needed.
3. Arrange the prosciutto-wrapped melon slices on a platter or board.
4. Slice the Mozzarella cheese into 1/4-inch thick slices and place on the platter.
5. Arrange the cherry tomatoes around the platter.
6. Sprinkle the fresh basil leaves over the platter.
7. Serve immediately and enjoy!

Tips:
- Choose a ripe melon for the best flavor and texture.
- Use high-quality prosciutto for the best flavor.
- Fresh Mozzarella is essential for this platter, as it has a creamy texture and mild flavor.
- You can also add other ingredients to the platter, such as grilled shrimp or sliced almonds, to add more flavor and texture.

7. Italian Delight

Ingredients:
- Prosciutto-wrapped Mozzarella (8 oz, 6g carbs)
- Cherry tomatoes (1 cup, 5g carbs)
- Fresh figs (1 cup, 7g carbs)
- Arugula (1/4 cup, 1g carbs)

Total carbs: 19g

Instructions:
1. Slice the Mozzarella cheese into 1/4-inch thick slices.
2. Wrap each slice with a slice of prosciutto, securing with a toothpick if needed.
3. Arrange the prosciutto-wrapped Mozzarella slices on a platter or board.
4. Halve the cherry tomatoes and arrange around the platter.
5. Slice the fresh figs and arrange on the platter.
6. Sprinkle the arugula leaves over the platter.
7. Serve immediately and enjoy!

Tips:
- Use high-quality prosciutto and Mozzarella for the best flavor.
- Fresh figs add a sweet and jammy element to the platter.
- Arugula adds a peppery flavor and crunchy texture.

8. Spanish Delight

Ingredients:
- Jaméno ibérico-wrapped melon (4-6 slices, 5g carbs)
- Manchego cheese (8 oz, 6g carbs)
- Grapes (1 cup, 6g carbs)
- Fresh rosemary (1/4 cup, 1g carbs)

Total carbs: 18g

Instructions:
1. Cut the melon into 1-inch thick slices.
2. Wrap each melon slice with a slice of Jamón ibérico, securing with a toothpick if needed.
3. Arrange the Jamón ibérico-wrapped melon slices on a platter or board.
4. Slice the Manchego cheese into 1/4-inch thick slices and place on the platter.
5. Arrange the grapes around the platter.
6. Sprinkle the fresh rosemary leaves over the platter.
7. Serve immediately and enjoy!

Tips:
- Jamón ibérico is a cured ham from Spain, known for its rich flavor and crunchy texture.
- Manchego cheese is a semi-firm cheese from Spain, with a nutty and slightly sweet flavor.
- Fresh rosemary adds a herbaceous and fragrant flavor to the platter.

9. Caprese Skewers

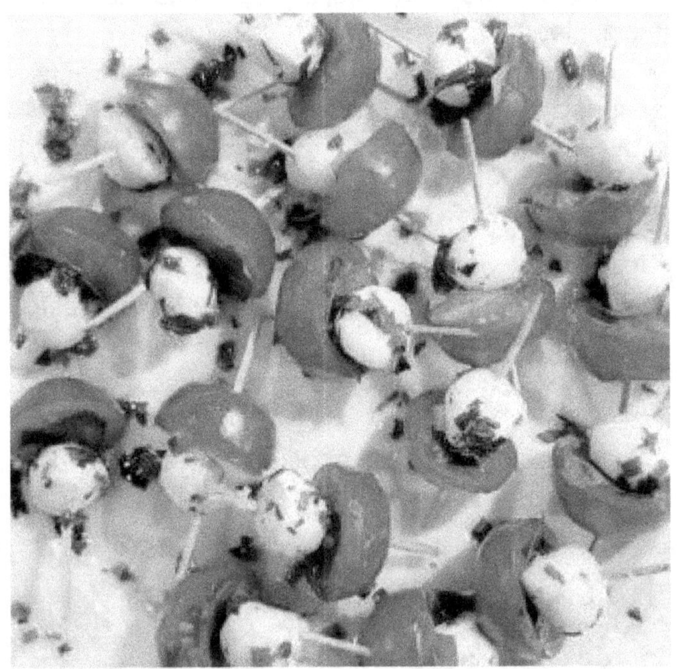

Ingredients:
- Fresh Mozzarella (8 oz, 6g carbs)
- Cherry tomatoes (1 cup, 5g carbs)
- Fresh basil (1/4 cup, 1g carbs)
- Prosciutto-wrapped skewers (4-6 skewers, 5g carbs)

Total carbs: 17g

Instructions:
1. Slice the Mozzarella cheese into 1-inch thick slices.
2. Halve the cherry tomatoes.

3. Cut the fresh basil leaves into smaller pieces.
4. Thread a cherry tomato, a Mozzarella slice, and a basil leaf onto a toothpick.
5. Wrap a slice of prosciutto around the skewer, securing with a toothpick if needed.
6. Repeat with the remaining ingredients.
7. Serve immediately and enjoy!

Tips:
- Use high-quality Mozzarella cheese for the best flavor.
- Fresh basil adds a bright and herbaceous flavor to the skewers.
- Prosciutto adds a salty and crunchy element to the skewers.

10. Gourmet Bites

Ingredients:
- Prosciutto-wrapped cantaloupe (4-6 slices, 5g carbs)
- Mozzarella and cherry tomato skewers (4-6 skewers, 5g carbs)
- Grilled shrimp (4-6 shrimp, 0g carbs)
- Fresh parsley (1/4 cup, 1g carbs)

Total carbs: 11g

Instructions:
1. Cut the cantaloupe into 1-inch thick slices.
2. Wrap each cantaloupe slice with a slice of prosciutto, securing with a toothpick if needed.

3. Thread a cherry tomato and a Mozzarella slice
onto a toothpick.
4. Grill the shrimp until pink and cooked through.
5. Arrange the prosciutto-wrapped cantaloupe,
Mozzarella and cherry tomato skewers, and grilled
shrimp on a platter.
6. Sprinkle the fresh parsley leaves over the platter.
7. Serve immediately and enjoy!

Tips:
- Use high-quality prosciutto and Mozzarella
cheese for the best flavor.
- Grilled shrimp add a protein-packed and flavorful
element to the platter.
- Fresh parsley adds a bright and herbaceous flavor
to the platter.

11. Flaxseed Crackers

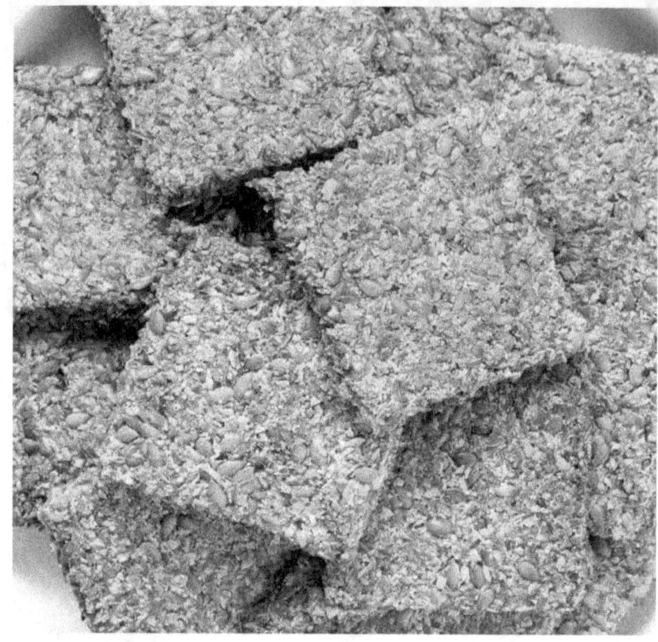

Ingredients:

- 1 cup ground flaxseed
- 1/2 cup water
- 1/4 teaspoon salt
- Optional: herbs and spices for flavor (e.g., garlic powder, dried rosemary, or sesame seeds)

Instructions:

1. Preheat your oven to 350°F (180°C). Line a baking sheet with parchment paper.
2. In a bowl, mix together the ground flaxseed and salt.

3. Gradually add in the water, stirring until the mixture forms a dough.
4. Knead the dough for about 5 minutes until it becomes pliable and smooth.
5. Divide the dough into 2-3 equal portions, depending on how large you want your crackers to be.
6. Roll out each portion into a thin sheet, about 1/8 inch thick.
7. Cut into desired shapes using a cookie cutter or a knife.
8. Place the crackers on the prepared baking sheet, leaving about 1 inch of space between each cracker.
9. Bake for 15-20 minutes or until the crackers are lightly golden and crispy.
10. Remove from the oven and let cool completely on the baking sheet.
11. Store in an airtight container for up to 5 days.

Tips:
- Make sure to use ground flaxseed, not whole flaxseeds.
- If the dough is too sticky, add a bit more flaxseed. If it's too dry, add a bit more water.
- You can flavor the crackers with herbs and spices before baking for extra taste.

12. Almond Flour Crackers

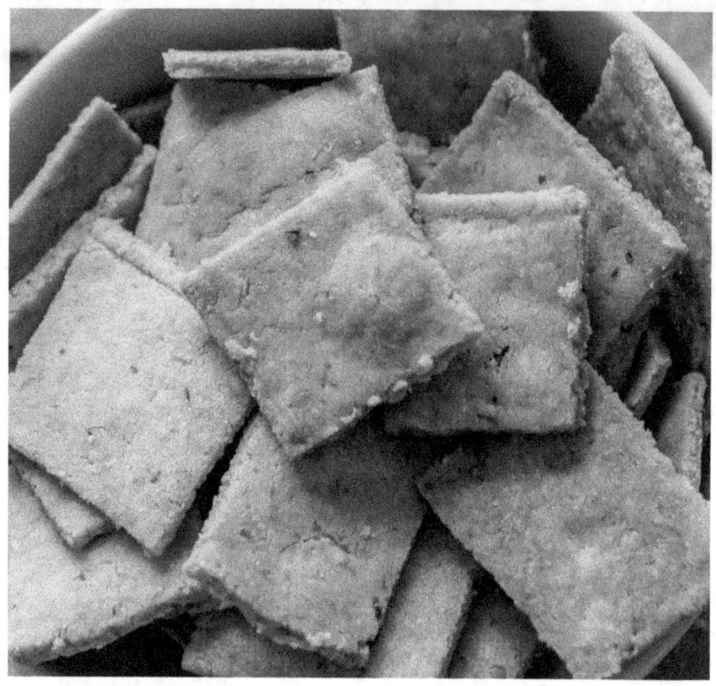

Ingredients:
- 2 cups almond flour
- 1/4 cup coconut flour
- 1/4 cup granulated sweetener (e.g., Swerve or Erythritol)
- 1/2 teaspoon salt
- 1/4 teaspoon baking soda
- 1/2 cup unsalted butter, melted
- 1 large egg
- Optional: herbs and spices for flavor (e.g., garlic powder, dried rosemary, or sesame seeds)

Instructions:
1. Preheat your oven to 350°F (180°C). Line a baking sheet with parchment paper.
2. In a large bowl, combine almond flour, coconut flour, sweetener, salt, and baking soda.
3. Mix in the melted butter and egg until a dough forms.
4. Knead the dough for about 5 minutes until it becomes pliable and smooth.
5. Divide the dough into 2-3 equal portions, depending on how large you want your crackers to be.
6. Roll out each portion into a thin sheet, about 1/8 inch thick.
7. Cut into desired shapes using a cookie cutter or a knife.
8. Place the crackers on the prepared baking sheet, leaving about 1 inch of space between each cracker.
9. Bake for 15-20 minutes or until the crackers are lightly golden and crispy.
10. Remove from the oven and let cool completely on the baking sheet.
11. Store in an airtight container for up to 5 days.

Tips:
- Make sure to use almond flour, not sliced almonds.
- If the dough is too sticky, add a bit more almond flour. If it's too dry, add a bit more egg.
- You can flavor the crackers with herbs and spices before baking for extra taste.

13. Veggie Chips

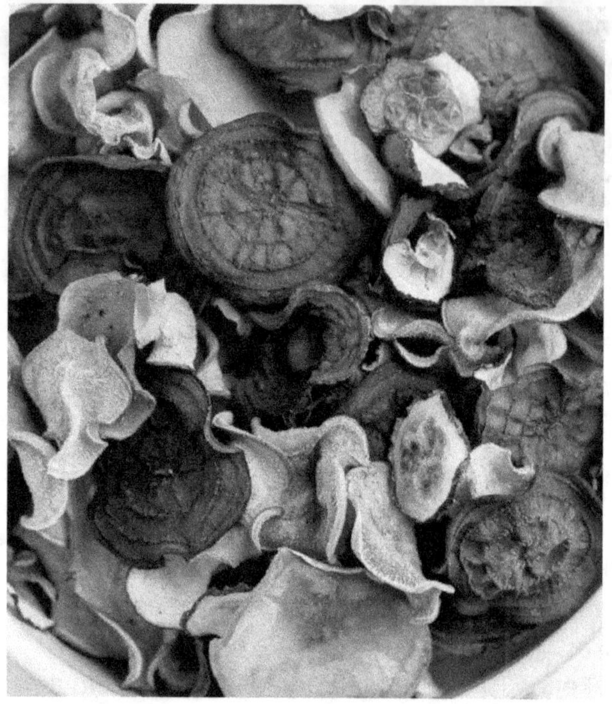

Ingredients:
- 2-3 cups mixed vegetables (e.g., kale, spinach, bell peppers, zucchini, carrots)
- 2 tablespoons olive oil
- Salt, to taste
- Optional: Additional seasonings (e.g., garlic powder, paprika, chili powder)

Instructions:
1. Preheat your oven to 250°F (120°C). Line a baking sheet with parchment paper.
2. Wash and dry the vegetables thoroughly.

3. Slice the vegetables into thin rounds or strips.
4. In a bowl, toss the vegetable slices with olive oil, salt, and any desired seasonings until evenly coated.
5. Spread the vegetable slices out in a single layer on the prepared baking sheet.
6. Bake for 1-2 hours or until the vegetables are crispy and golden brown, flipping halfway through.
7. Remove from the oven and let cool completely on the baking sheet.
8. Store in an airtight container for up to 24 hours.

Tips:
- Use a variety of colorful vegetables for a mix of flavors and textures.
- Keep an eye on the veggie chips during baking, as they can go from perfect to burnt quickly.
- Enjoy your crispy and healthy veggie chips as a low-carb snack!

14. Cheese Crisps

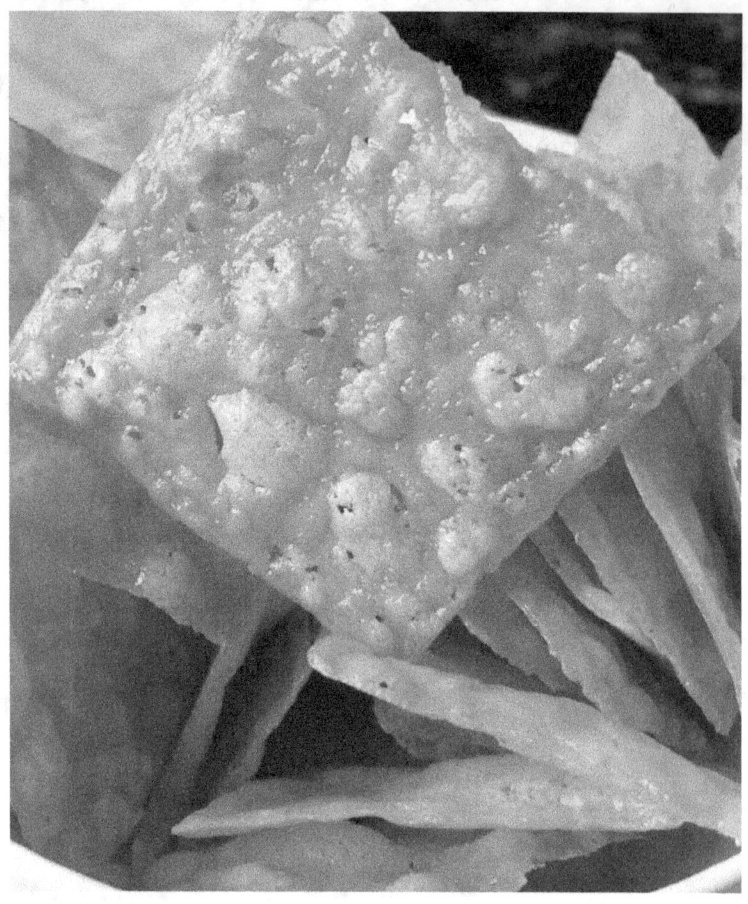

Ingredients:
- 1 cup shredded cheese (e.g., cheddar, mozzarella, Parmesan, or a mix)
- 1/4 cup almond flour
- 1/4 cup coconut flour
- 1/2 teaspoon salt
- 1/4 teaspoon baking soda

- 1/2 cup unsalted butter, melted
- Optional: herbs and spices for flavor (e.g., garlic powder, dried rosemary, or paprika)

Instructions:
1. Preheat your oven to 350°F (180°C). Line a baking sheet with parchment paper.
2. In a bowl, mix together the shredded cheese, almond flour, coconut flour, salt, and baking soda.
3. Add the melted butter and mix until a dough forms.
4. Roll out the dough on a floured surface to about 1/8 inch thickness.
5. Cut into desired shapes using a cookie cutter or a knife.
6. Place the cheese crisps on the prepared baking sheet, leaving about 1 inch of space between each cracker.
7. Bake for 10-12 minutes or until the cheese crisps are golden brown and crispy.
8. Remove from the oven and let cool completely on the baking sheet.
9. Store in an airtight container for up to 5 days.

Tips:
- Use a variety of cheeses for a unique flavor profile.
- Keep an eye on the cheese crisps during baking, as they can go from perfect to burnt quickly.
- Enjoy your crispy and delicious cheese crisps as a low-carb snack!

15. Pork Rinds

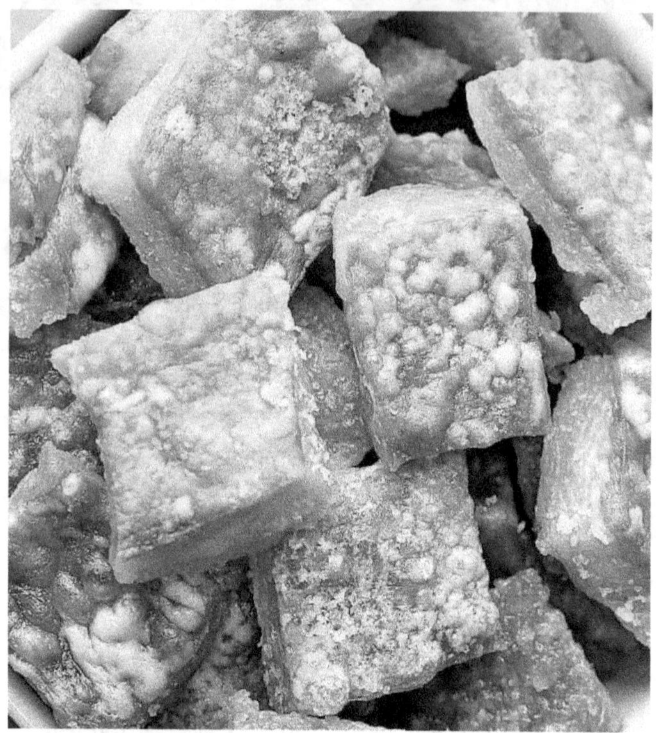

Ingredients:
- 2 cups pork skin, cut into small pieces
- 1/4 cup olive oil
- 1/2 teaspoon salt
- 1/4 teaspoon black pepper
- 1/4 teaspoon garlic powder (optional)
- 1/4 teaspoon paprika (optional)

Instructions:
1. Preheat your oven to 400°F (200°C). Line a baking sheet with parchment paper.

2. In a bowl, mix together the pork skin pieces, olive oil, salt, black pepper, garlic powder, and paprika (if using).
3. Spread the pork skin mixture out in a single layer on the prepared baking sheet.
4. Bake for 20-25 minutes or until the pork skin is crispy and golden brown, flipping halfway through.
5. Remove from the oven and let cool completely on the baking sheet.
6. Store in an airtight container for up to 5 days.

Tips:
- Use pork skin with the fat layer intact for the crispiest results.
- Keep an eye on the pork rinds during baking, as they can go from perfect to burnt quickly.
- Enjoy your crispy and delicious pork rinds as a low-carb snack!

Note: You can also make pork rinds in a deep fryer or a skillet on the stovetop, but baking is a healthier and easier option.

Soups And Salads

1. Creamy Tomato Soup

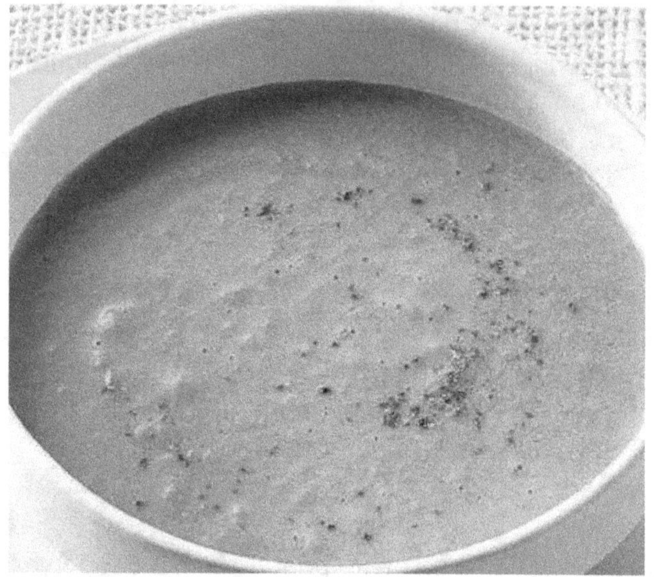

Ingredients:
- 3 cups fresh tomatoes, chopped
- 2 tablespoons butter
- 1 onion, chopped
- 3 cloves garlic, minced
- 1 cup chicken broth
- 1 cup heavy cream
- 1 teaspoon dried basil
- Salt and pepper, to taste

Instructions:
1. In a large pot, melt the butter over medium heat.

2. Add the chopped onion and cook until softened, about 5 minutes.
3. Add the minced garlic and cook for an additional minute.
4. Add the chopped tomatoes, chicken broth, and dried basil.
5. Bring the mixture to a boil, then reduce the heat and simmer for 15-20 minutes.
6. Use an immersion blender to puree the soup until smooth.
7. Stir in the heavy cream and season with salt and pepper to taste.
8. Serve hot and enjoy!

Note: You can also use canned tomatoes if fresh tomatoes are not available. Just be sure to choose a low-carb option.

2. Chicken And Vegetable Broth

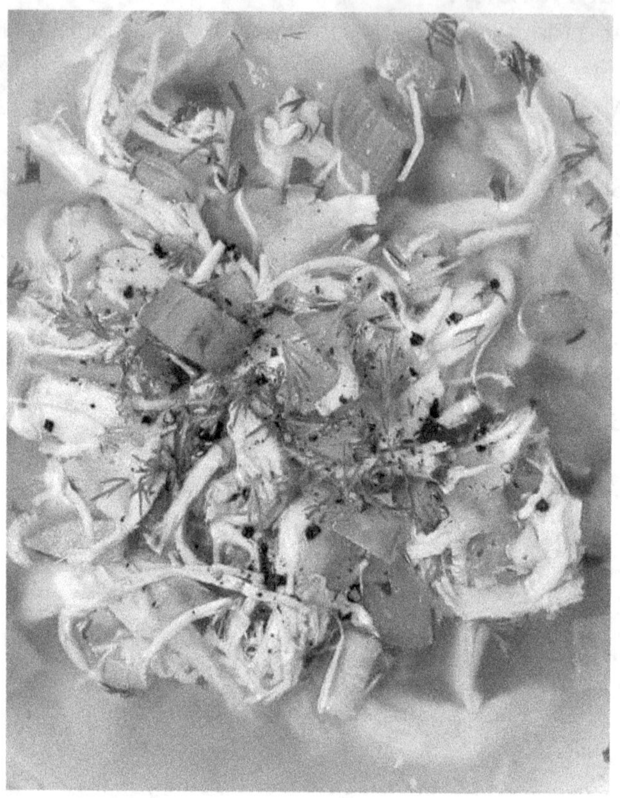

Ingredients:
- 1 whole chicken (3-4 lbs), cut into pieces
- 4 cups water
- 2 carrots, chopped
- 2 celery stalks, chopped
- 2 cloves garlic, minced
- 1 large onion, chopped
- 2 sprigs fresh parsley
- Salt and pepper, to taste

Instructions:
1. In a large pot, combine the chicken pieces,
water, chopped carrots, celery, garlic, and onion.
2. Bring the mixture to a boil, then reduce the heat
and simmer for 30-40 minutes or until the chicken is
cooked through.
3. Remove the chicken from the pot and let it cool.
4. Strain the broth through a fine-mesh sieve into a
clean pot, discarding the solids.
5. Add the chopped parsley and season with salt
and pepper to taste.
6. Serve hot and enjoy!

Note: You can also use a slow cooker or Instant
Pot to make this recipe. Just adjust the cooking
time accordingly.

3. Cauliflower Soup

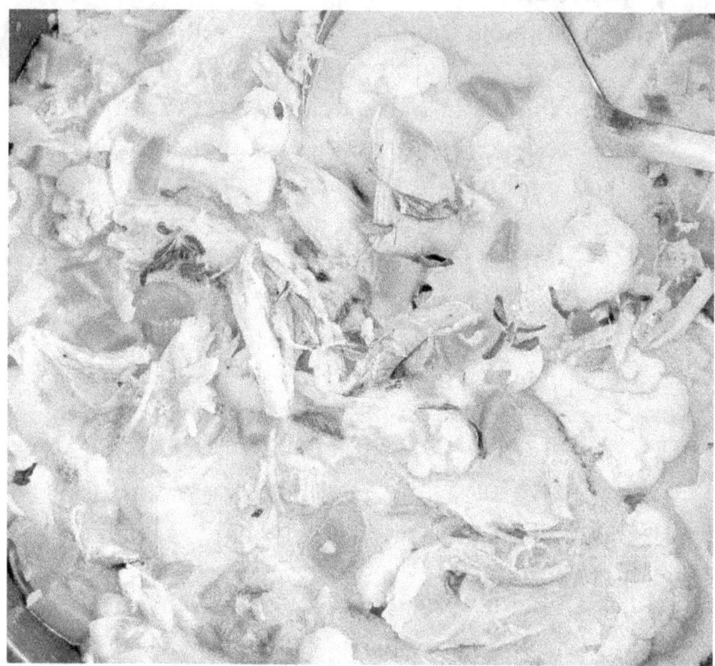

Ingredients:
- 1 head cauliflower, broken into florets
- 2 tablespoons butter
- 1 onion, chopped
- 3 cloves garlic, minced
- 1 cup chicken broth
- 1 cup heavy cream
- Salt and pepper, to taste
- Optional: nutmeg, paprika, or other spices of your choice

Instructions:
1. In a large pot, melt the butter over medium heat.

2. Add the chopped onion and cook until softened, about 5 minutes.
3. Add the minced garlic and cook for an additional minute.
4. Add the cauliflower florets and cook until they start to soften, about 5 minutes.
5. Pour in the chicken broth and bring the mixture to a boil.
6. Reduce the heat and simmer until the cauliflower is tender, about 15-20 minutes.
7. Stir in the heavy cream and season with salt, pepper, and any desired spices.
8. Serve hot and enjoy!

Note: You can also add other ingredients like cooked bacon, diced ham, or grated cheese to give the soup extra flavor.

4. Keto Cream Of Mushroom Soup

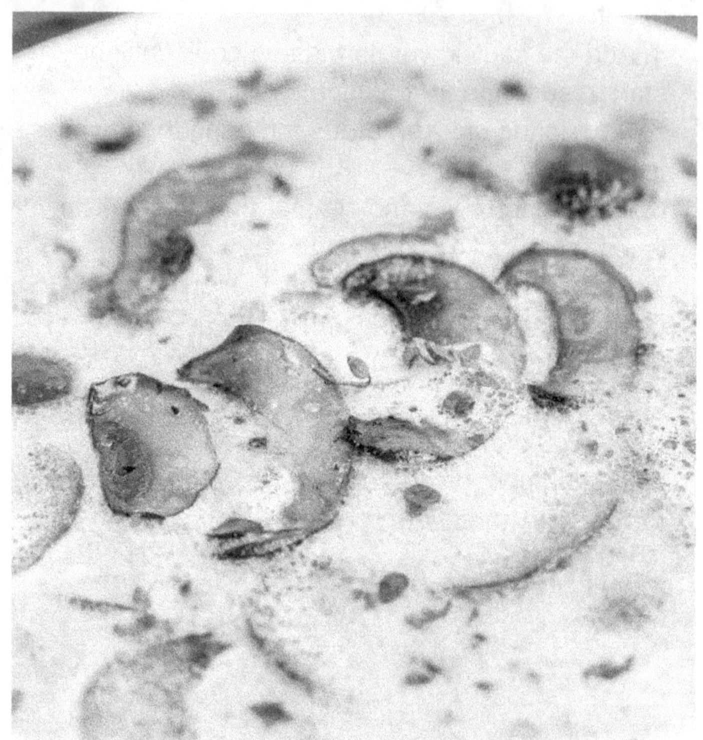

Ingredients:
- 2 cups mixed mushrooms (button, cremini, shiitake), sliced
- 2 tablespoons butter
- 1 onion, chopped
- 3 cloves garlic, minced
- 1 cup chicken broth
- 1 cup heavy cream
- 1/2 cup grated Parmesan cheese

- Salt and pepper, to taste
- Fresh parsley, chopped (optional)

Instructions:
1. In a large pot, melt the butter over medium heat.
2. Add the chopped onion and cook until softened, about 5 minutes.
3. Add the minced garlic and cook for an additional minute.
4. Add the sliced mushrooms and cook until they release their moisture and start to brown, about 5-7 minutes.
5. Pour in the chicken broth and bring the mixture to a simmer.
6. Reduce the heat and let cook for 10-15 minutes or until the mushrooms are tender.
7. Stir in the heavy cream and Parmesan cheese until melted and smooth.
8. Season with salt and pepper to taste.
9. Serve hot, garnished with chopped parsley if desired.

Note: Make sure to choose a low-carb chicken broth and heavy cream to keep the soup keto-friendly.

5. Low-Carb Chicken Noodle Soup

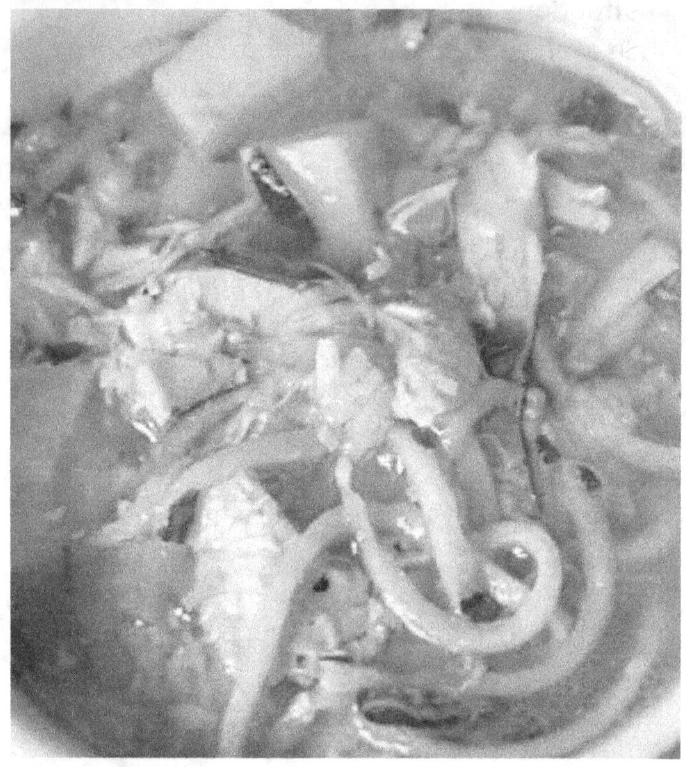

Ingredients:
- 1 pound boneless, skinless chicken breast or thighs
- 4 cups chicken broth (low-carb)
- 1 medium onion, chopped
- 2 cloves garlic, minced
- 2 cups zucchini noodles (zoodles) or low-carb noodles
- 1 teaspoon dried basil

- 1 teaspoon dried oregano
- Salt and pepper, to taste

Instructions:
1. In a large pot, sauté the chopped onion and minced garlic in a little bit of oil until softened.
2. Add the chicken and cook until browned on all sides.
3. Pour in the chicken broth, dried basil, and dried oregano.
4. Bring the mixture to a boil, then reduce the heat and simmer for 10-15 minutes or until the chicken is cooked through.
5. Add the zucchini noodles or low-carb noodles and cook for an additional 2-3 minutes.
6. Season with salt and pepper to taste.
7. Serve hot and enjoy!

Note: You can use a low-carb noodle substitute like zucchini noodles, spaghetti squash, or shirataki noodles to keep the soup low in carbs.

6. Spinach And Artichoke Soup

Ingredients:
- 2 cups fresh spinach leaves
- 1 (14 oz) can artichoke hearts, drained and chopped
- 2 tablespoons butter
- 1 onion, chopped
- 3 cloves garlic, minced
- 1 cup chicken broth

- 1 cup heavy cream
- 1/2 cup grated Parmesan cheese
- Salt and pepper, to taste

Instructions:
1. In a large pot, melt the butter over medium heat.
2. Add the chopped onion and cook until softened, about 5 minutes.
3. Add the minced garlic and cook for an additional minute.
4. Add the chopped artichoke hearts, spinach leaves, chicken broth, and heavy cream.
5. Bring the mixture to a simmer and let cook for 10-15 minutes or until the spinach is wilted.
6. Use an immersion blender to puree the soup until smooth.
7. Stir in the Parmesan cheese until melted and smooth.
8. Season with salt and pepper to taste.
9. Serve hot and enjoy!

Note: You can also add other ingredients like cooked bacon, diced ham, or a sprinkle of red pepper flakes to give the soup extra flavor.

7. Roasted Vegetable Soup

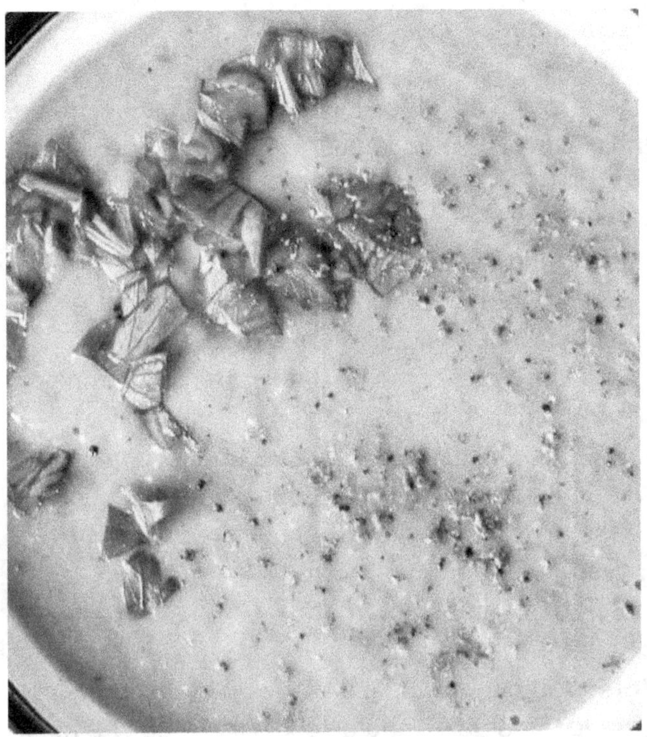

Ingredients:
- 2 tablespoons olive oil
- 1 onion, chopped
- 3 cloves garlic, minced
- 3 carrots, peeled and chopped
- 3 celery stalks, chopped
- 2 potatoes, peeled and chopped
- 2 cups mixed vegetables (such as zucchini, bell peppers, and tomatoes)
- 4 cups vegetable broth
- 1 teaspoon dried thyme

- Salt and pepper, to taste

Instructions:
1. Preheat the oven to 425°F (220°C).
2. In a large bowl, toss together the chopped onion, garlic, carrots, celery, potatoes, and mixed vegetables.
3. Drizzle with olive oil and season with salt, pepper, and thyme.
4. Spread the vegetables on a baking sheet and roast for 30-40 minutes or until tender.
5. In a large pot, combine the roasted vegetables and vegetable broth.
6. Bring the mixture to a simmer and let cook for 10-15 minutes or until heated through.
7. Use an immersion blender to puree the soup until smooth.
8. Serve hot and enjoy!

Note: You can customize the recipe by using your favorite vegetables and spices. Also, you can make it a creamy soup by adding heavy cream or coconut cream.

8. Creamy Asparagus Soup

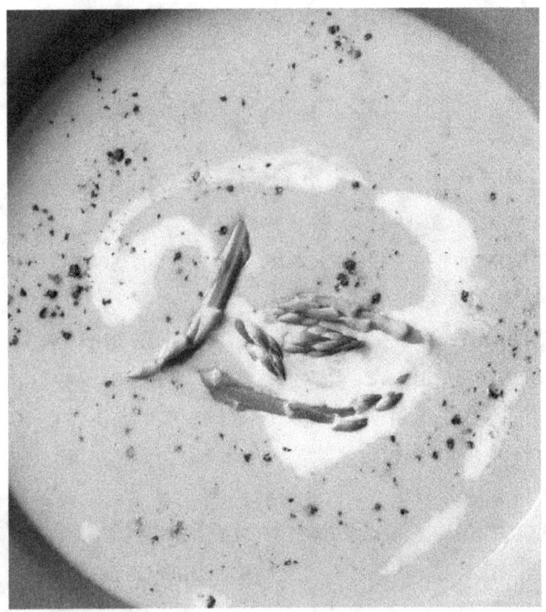

Ingredients:
- 2 pounds fresh asparagus, trimmed
- 2 tablespoons butter
- 1 onion, chopped
- 3 cloves garlic, minced
- 1 cup chicken broth
- 1 cup heavy cream
- 1/2 cup grated Parmesan cheese
- Salt and pepper, to taste

Instructions:
1. In a large pot, melt the butter over medium heat.
2. Add the chopped onion and cook until softened, about 5 minutes.

3. Add the minced garlic and cook for an additional minute.
4. Add the asparagus and cook until tender, about 5-7 minutes.
5. Pour in the chicken broth and bring the mixture to a simmer.
6. Reduce the heat and let cook for 10-15 minutes or until the asparagus is very tender.
7. Use an immersion blender to puree the soup until smooth.
8. Stir in the heavy cream and Parmesan cheese until melted and smooth.
9. Season with salt and pepper to taste.
10. Serve hot and enjoy!

Note: You can also add other ingredients like cooked bacon, diced ham, or a sprinkle of paprika to give the soup extra flavor.

9. Classic Greek Salad

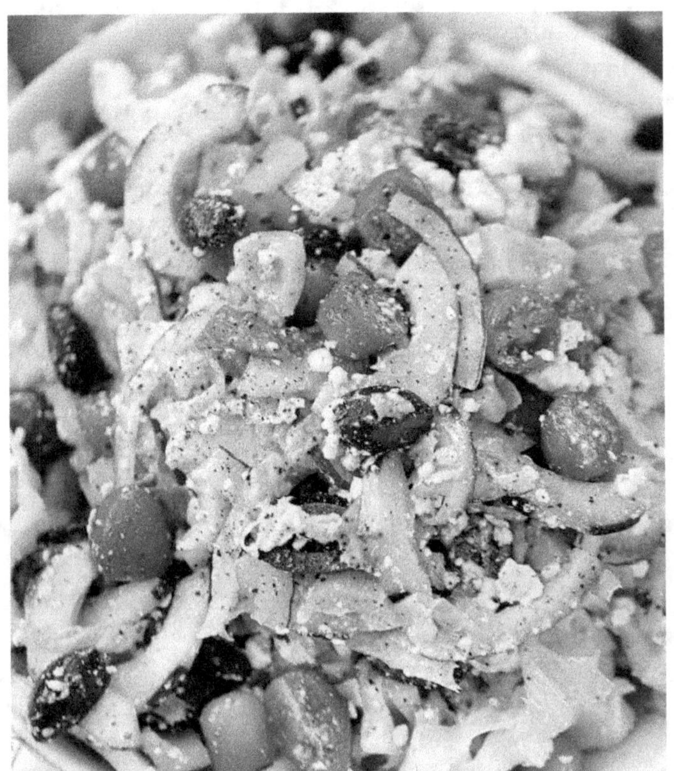

Ingredients:
- 4-6 cups mixed greens (romaine, arugula, spinach)
- 1 large tomato, diced
- 1 large cucumber, peeled and sliced
- 1 cup Kalamata olives, pitted
- 1 cup crumbled feta cheese
- 1/4 cup red onion, thinly sliced
- 2 tbsp. extra-virgin olive oil
- 2 tbsp. red wine vinegar

- Salt and pepper, to taste

Instructions:
1. In a large bowl, combine the mixed greens, tomato, cucumber, olives, feta cheese, and red onion.
2. In a small bowl, whisk together the olive oil and red wine vinegar.
3. Pour the dressing over the salad and toss to combine.
4. Season with salt and pepper to taste.
5. Serve immediately and enjoy!

Note: You can customize the recipe to your liking by adding other ingredients such as grilled chicken, bell peppers, or capers.

10. Spinach And Strawberry Salad

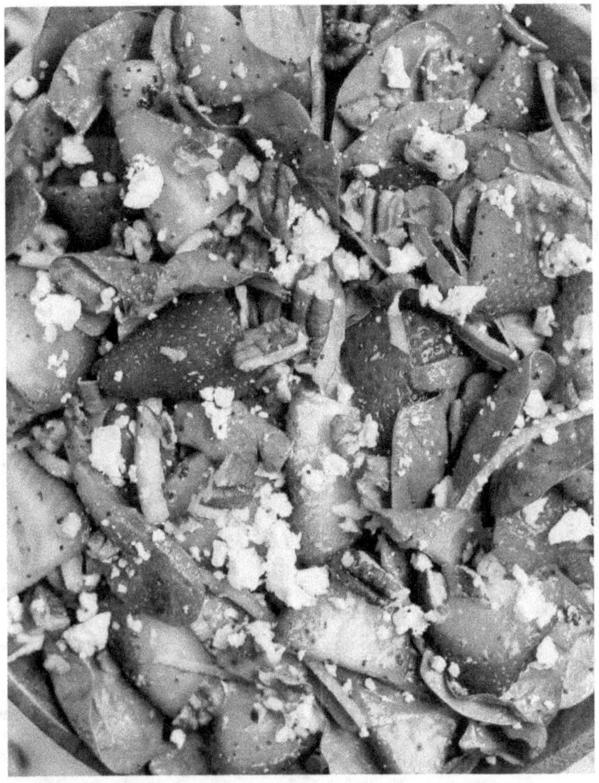

Ingredients:
- 4 cups fresh baby spinach leaves
- 1 pint fresh strawberries, hulled and sliced
- 1/2 cup crumbled feta cheese
- 1/4 cup chopped pecans or walnuts
- 1/4 cup olive oil
- 2 tbsp. balsamic vinegar
- Salt and pepper, to taste

Instructions:

1. In a large bowl, combine the spinach leaves, strawberry slices, feta cheese, and chopped nuts.
2. In a small bowl, whisk together the olive oil and balsamic vinegar.
3. Pour the dressing over the salad and toss to combine.
4. Season with salt and pepper to taste.
5. Serve immediately and enjoy!

Note: You can customize the recipe by adding other ingredients like grilled chicken, avocado, or red onion. Also, you can use other types of cheese like goat cheese or parmesan.

11. Keto Cobb Salad

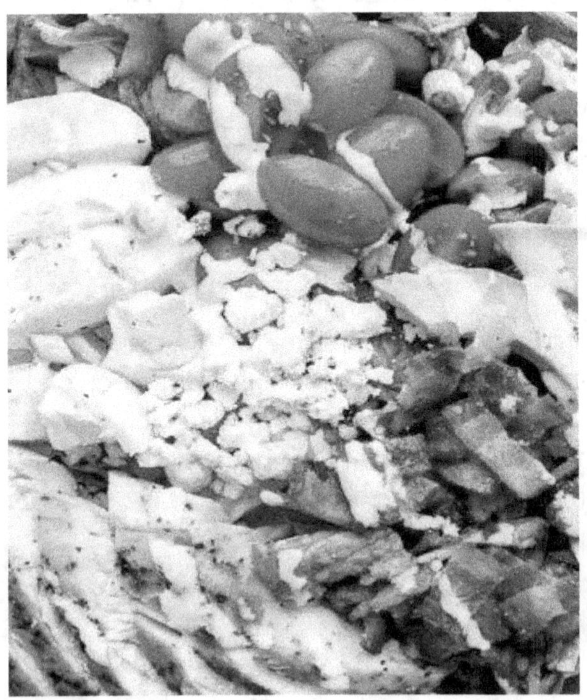

Ingredients:

- 4 cups mixed greens (lettuce, spinach, arugula)
- 1 cup cooked chicken breast, diced
- 1/2 cup avocado, diced
- 1/2 cup bacon, cooked and crumbled
- 1/2 cup blue cheese, crumbled
- 1/4 cup chopped hard-boiled egg
- 1/4 cup olive oil
- 2 tbsp. lemon juice
- Salt and pepper, to taste

Instructions:

1. In a large bowl, combine the mixed greens, chicken breast, avocado, bacon, blue cheese, and hard-boiled egg.
2. In a small bowl, whisk together the olive oil and lemon juice.
3. Pour the dressing over the salad and toss to combine.
4. Season with salt and pepper to taste.
5. Serve immediately and enjoy!

Note: To make this salad keto-friendly, use a sugar-free dressing and be mindful of the portion sizes to keep the carb count low. Also, you can customize the recipe by adding other ingredients like tomatoes or spinach.

12. Low-Carb Chicken Caesar Salad

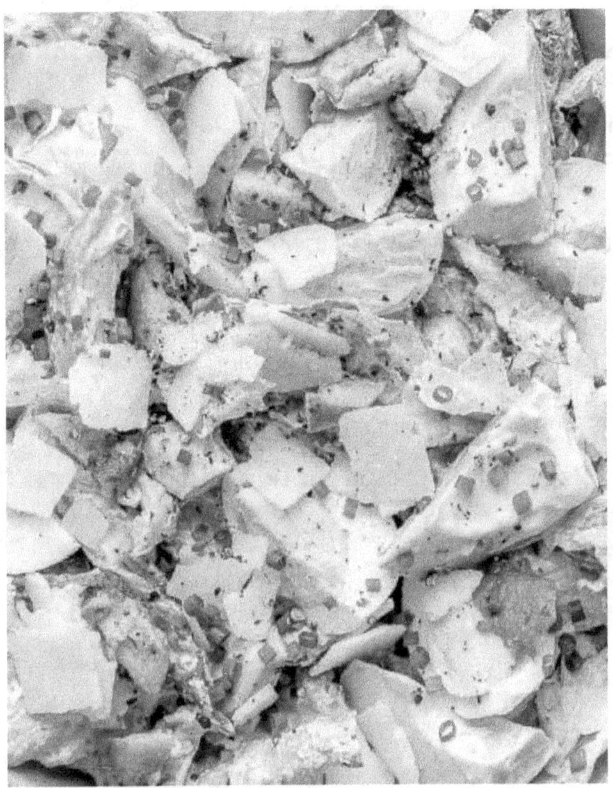

Ingredients:
- 4 cups romaine lettuce, chopped
- 1 cup cooked chicken breast, diced
- 1/2 cup parmesan cheese, shaved
- 1/4 cup homemade Caesar dressing (made with olive oil, lemon juice, egg, garlic, and anchovy paste)
- 1/4 cup chopped bacon (optional)

Instructions:
1. In a large bowl, combine the romaine lettuce, chicken breast, and parmesan cheese.
2. Drizzle the homemade Caesar dressing over the salad and toss to combine.
3. Top with chopped bacon, if desired.
4. Serve immediately and enjoy!

Note: To make this salad low-carb, use a sugar-free Caesar dressing and be mindful of the portion sizes to keep the carb count low. Also, you can customize the recipe by adding other ingredients like avocado or tomatoes.

Here is a simple recipe for homemade Caesar dressing

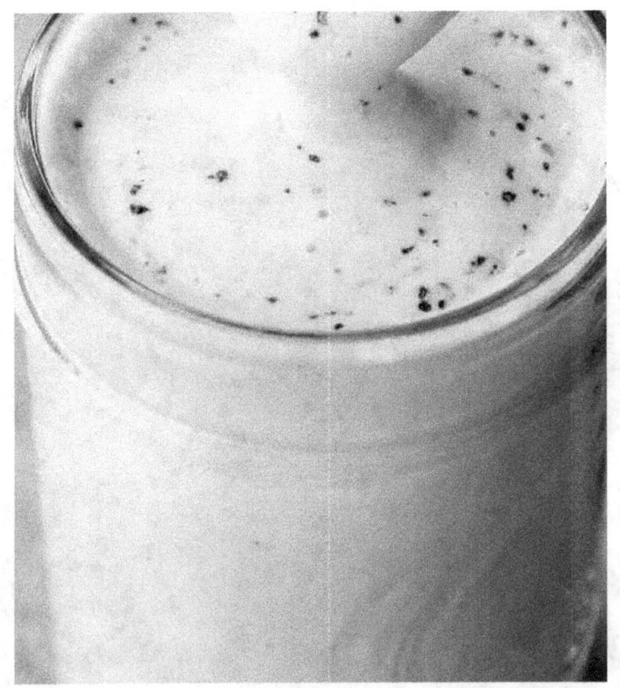

Ingredients:
- 2 cloves garlic, minced
- 2 anchovy filets, minced
- 1 egg
- 2 tbsp. freshly squeezed lemon juice
- 1 cup olive oil
- Salt and pepper, to taste

Instructions:
1. Blend all ingredients except olive oil in a blender or food processor.
2. Slowly pour in olive oil while blending until smooth.
3. Taste and adjust seasoning as needed.

13. Caprese Salad

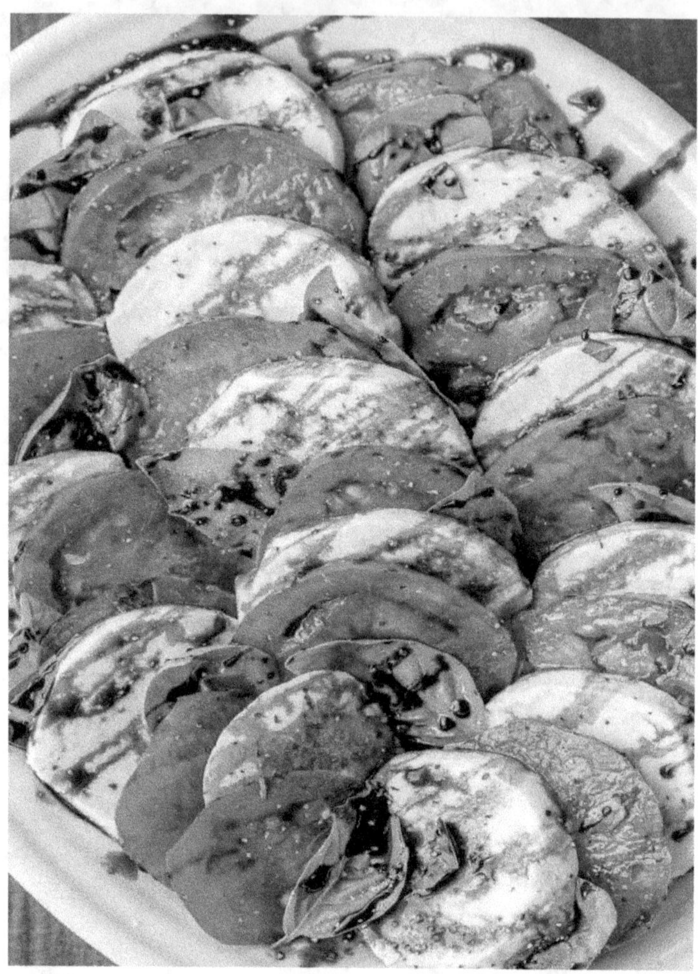

Ingredients:
- 3 large tomatoes, sliced
- 8 ounces fresh mozzarella cheese, sliced
- 1/4 cup extra-virgin olive oil
- 2 tablespoons balsamic vinegar

- 1/4 cup fresh basil leaves, chopped
- Salt and pepper, to taste

Instructions:
1. Arrange the tomato slices on a large plate or platter.
2. Top each tomato slice with a slice of mozzarella cheese.
3. Drizzle the olive oil and balsamic vinegar over the salad.
4. Sprinkle the chopped basil leaves over the top.
5. Season with salt and pepper to taste.
6. Serve immediately and enjoy!

Note: This salad is best made with fresh, high-quality ingredients, as it allows the natural flavors to shine through. You can also add other ingredients like grilled chicken or prosciutto to make it more substantial.

14. Taco Salad

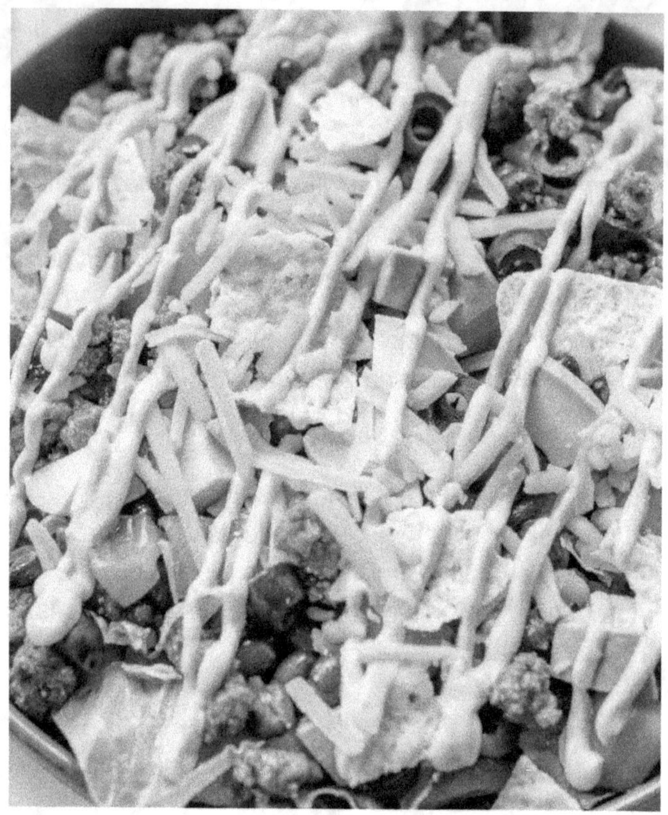

Ingredients:
- 4 cups mixed greens (lettuce, spinach, arugula)
- 1 cup cooked ground beef (or ground turkey, chicken, or beans for a vegetarian option)
- 1 cup tortilla chips, crushed
- 1 cup shredded cheese (cheddar or Monterey Jack work well)
- 1 can (14.5 oz) diced tomatoes, drained
- 1/4 cup chopped red onion

- 1/4 cup chopped cilantro
- 2 tbsp. olive oil
- 1 tbsp. lime juice
- 1 tsp. taco seasoning
- Salt and pepper, to taste

Instructions:

1. In a large bowl, combine the mixed greens, ground beef, tortilla chips, shredded cheese, diced tomatoes, red onion, and cilantro.
2. In a small bowl, whisk together the olive oil, lime juice, and taco seasoning.
3. Pour the dressing over the salad and toss to combine.
4. Season with salt and pepper to taste.
5. Serve immediately and enjoy!

Note: You can customize this recipe to your liking by adding other ingredients like diced bell peppers, jalapenos, or avocado. Also, you can use store-bought taco seasoning or make your own blend with chili powder, cumin, and paprika.

15. Chicken And Avocado Salad

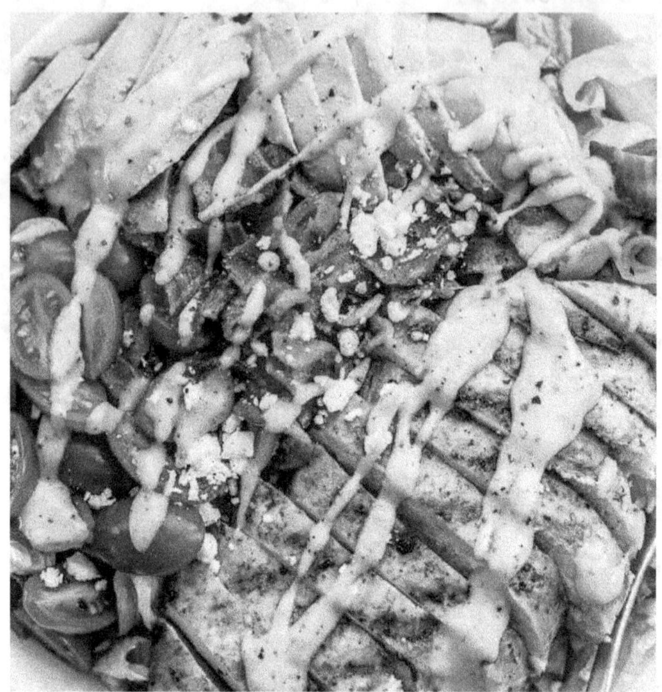

Ingredients:

- 4 cups mixed greens (lettuce, spinach, arugula)
- 1 cup cooked chicken breast, diced
- 1 ripe avocado, diced
- 1/2 cup cherry tomatoes, halved
- 1/4 cup red onion, thinly sliced
- 1/4 cup crumbled feta cheese (optional)
- 2 tbsp. olive oil
- 1 tbsp. lemon juice
- Salt and pepper, to taste

Instructions:

1. In a large bowl, combine the mixed greens, chicken breast, avocado, cherry tomatoes, and red onion.
2. In a small bowl, whisk together the olive oil and lemon juice.
3. Pour the dressing over the salad and toss to combine.
4. Top with crumbled feta cheese, if desired.
5. Season with salt and pepper to taste.
6. Serve immediately and enjoy!

Note: You can customize this recipe to your liking by adding other ingredients like bacon, nuts, or diced bell peppers. Also, you can use different types of cheese like parmesan or goat cheese instead of feta.

Entrees

1. Grilled Steak With Roasted Vegetables

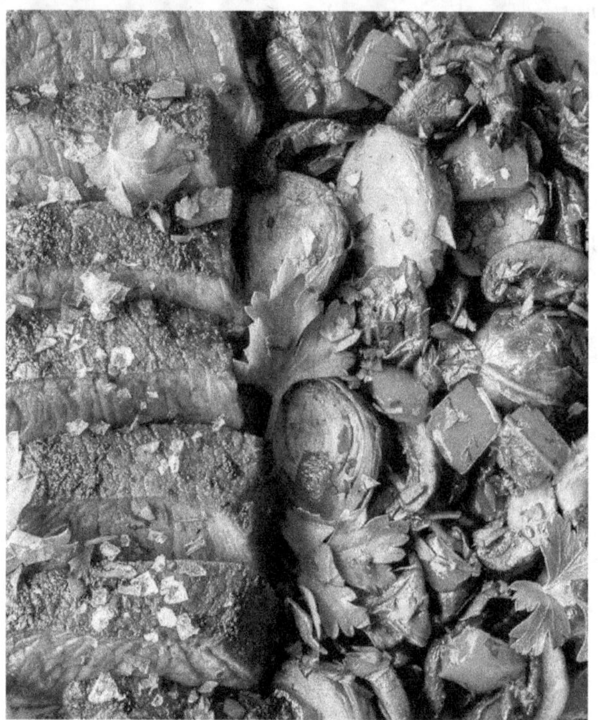

Ingredients:
- 1.5 lbs steak (Ribeye or Sirloin work well)
- 2 tbsp olive oil
- 2 cloves garlic, minced
- 1 tsp dried thyme
- 1 tsp paprika
- Salt and pepper, to taste

- 4 cups mixed vegetables (such as broccoli, cauliflower, Brussels sprouts, and red onion)

Instructions:
1. Preheat the grill to medium-high heat.
2. In a small bowl, mix together olive oil, garlic, thyme, paprika, salt, and pepper.
3. Brush the mixture on both sides of the steak.
4. Grill the steak for 5-7 minutes per side, or until it reaches your desired level of doneness.
5. Meanwhile, toss the vegetables in olive oil, salt, and pepper, and spread on a baking sheet.
6. Roast in the oven at 425°F (220°C) for 20-25 minutes, or until tender and lightly browned.
7. Serve the steak with the roasted vegetables and enjoy!

Note: You can adjust the vegetables to your liking and add other low-carb options like mushrooms or bell peppers. Also, make sure to check the steak's internal temperature to ensure it reaches a safe minimum internal temperature of 135°F (57°C) for medium-rare.

2. Beef And Mushroom Stroganoff

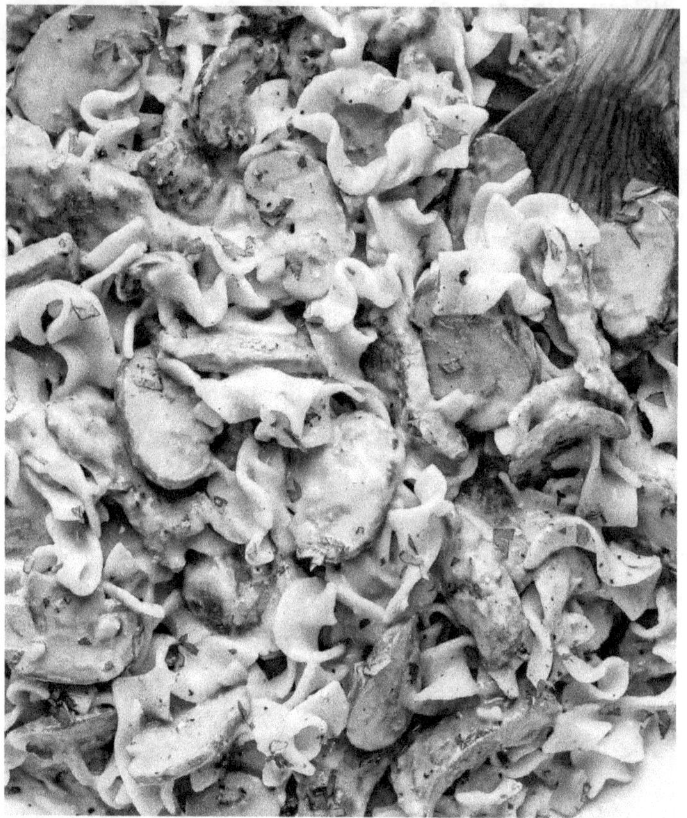

Ingredients:
- 1 lb beef strips (sirloin or ribeye work well)
- 2 cups mixed mushrooms (button, cremini, and shiitake)
- 2 tbsp butter
- 1 onion, finely chopped
- 2 cloves garlic, minced

- 1 cup beef broth
- 1/2 cup Greek yogurt
- 1 tsp Dijon mustard
- 1 tsp paprika
- Salt and pepper, to taste
- Fresh parsley, chopped (optional)

Instructions:
1. Cook the beef strips in butter until browned, then set aside.
2. In the same pan, sauté the mushrooms, onion, and garlic until tender.
3. Add beef broth, yogurt, mustard, paprika, salt, and pepper. Stir to combine.
4. Return the beef to the pan and simmer until coated in the sauce.
5. Serve hot, garnished with chopped parsley if desired.

Note: You can serve this dish with a side of sautéed spinach or roasted vegetables to keep it low-carb. Also, adjust the amount of beef broth and yogurt to achieve your desired level of creaminess.

3. Low-Carb Beef Tacos

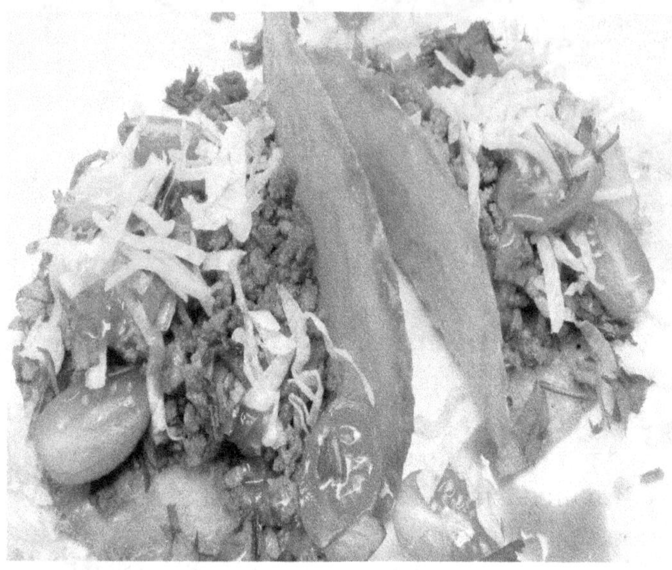

Ingredients:
- 1 lb ground beef
- 1/2 cup chopped onion
- 1/2 cup chopped bell pepper
- 2 cloves garlic, minced
- 1 packet taco seasoning (check the carb count)
- 8 low-carb taco shells (check the carb count)
- Shredded cheese, lettuce, avocado, sour cream, and any other desired toppings

Instructions:
1. Cook the ground beef in a skillet until browned, breaking it up into small pieces.
2. Add the onion, bell pepper, and garlic to the skillet and cook until tender.

3. Add the taco seasoning and cook according to the package instructions.
4. Warm the low-carb taco shells according to the package instructions.
5. Assemble the tacos with the beef mixture, cheese, lettuce, avocado, sour cream, and any other desired toppings.

Note: Make sure to check the carb count on the taco seasoning and low-carb taco shells to ensure they fit within your daily carb limit. Also, be mindful of the toppings you choose, as some may be higher in carbs.

4. Pork Chop With Apple And Onion

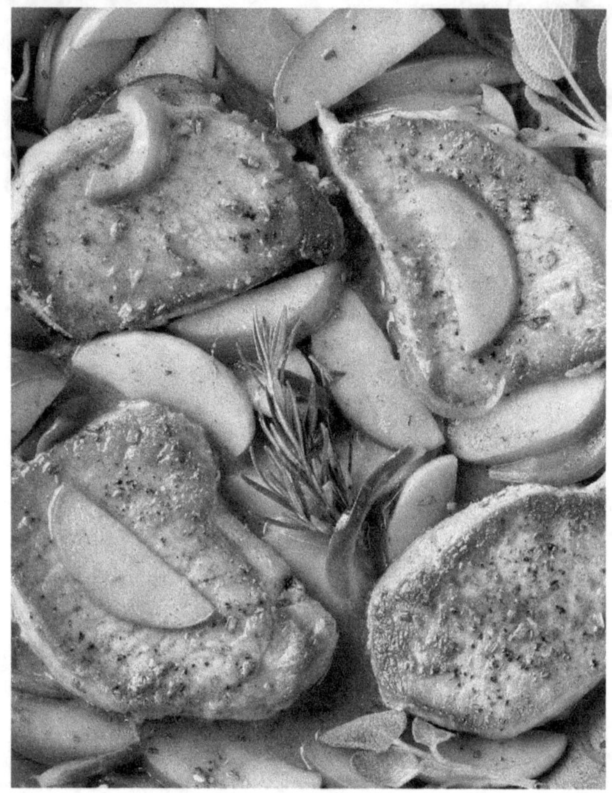

Ingredients:
- 4 pork chops (1-1.5 lbs)
- 2 apples, sliced
- 1 large onion, sliced
- 2 tbsp olive oil
- 1 tsp cinnamon
- 1 tsp nutmeg
- Salt and pepper, to taste

Instructions:
1. Preheat the oven to 400°F (200°C).
2. In a large skillet, heat olive oil over medium-high heat.
3. Sear the pork chops until browned, about 2-3 minutes per side.
4. Transfer the pork chops to a baking sheet and top with apple and onion slices.
5. Sprinkle cinnamon, nutmeg, salt, and pepper to taste.
6. Bake in the preheated oven for 20-25 minutes or until the pork chops reach an internal temperature of 145°F (63°C).
7. Serve hot and enjoy!

Note: You can adjust the amount of apples and onions to your liking, and also add other spices or herbs to the pork chops for extra flavor. This recipe is not only delicious but also low in carbs, making it a great option for a low-carb diet.

5. Cauliflower Fried Rice With Pork

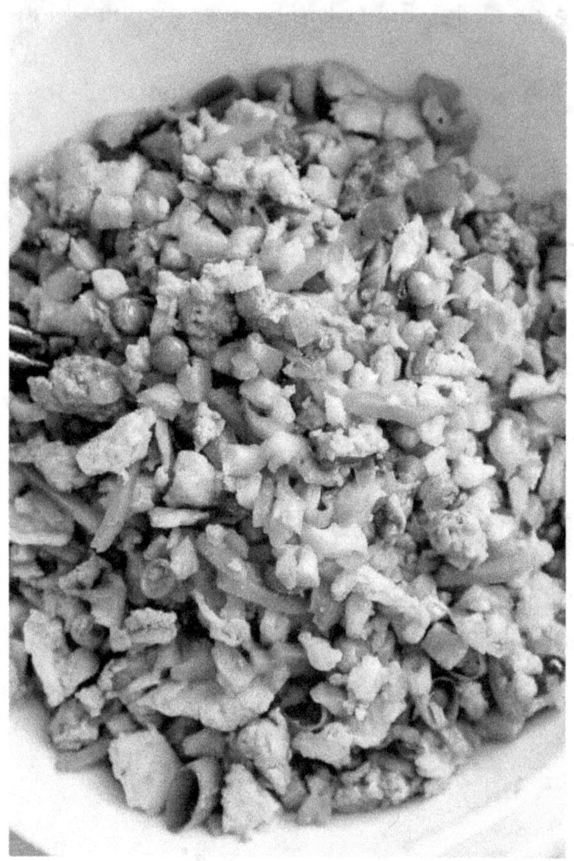

Ingredients:
- 1 head of cauliflower
- 1 lb ground pork
- 2 cups mixed vegetables (e.g., peas, carrots, corn)
- 2 tbsp coconut oil

- 2 cloves garlic, minced
- 1 tsp soy sauce
- 1 tsp oyster sauce (optional)
- Salt and pepper, to taste
- 2 eggs, beaten (optional)

Instructions:
1. Pulse cauliflower in a food processor until it resembles rice.
2. Cook the ground pork in a skillet until browned, breaking it up into small pieces.
3. Add mixed vegetables, coconut oil, garlic, soy sauce, and oyster sauce (if using) to the skillet. Cook until the vegetables are tender.
4. Add the cauliflower "rice" to the skillet and stir-fry until combined with the pork and vegetable mixture.
5. If using eggs, push the cauliflower mixture to one side of the skillet, crack in the eggs, and scramble them until cooked through. Then mix the eggs with the cauliflower mixture.
6. Season with salt and pepper to taste.
7. Serve hot and enjoy!

Note: This recipe is a low-carb version of traditional fried rice, using cauliflower instead of rice. You can customize it to your taste by adding other vegetables, spices, or protein sources like shrimp or chicken.

6. Chicken And Mushroom Crepes

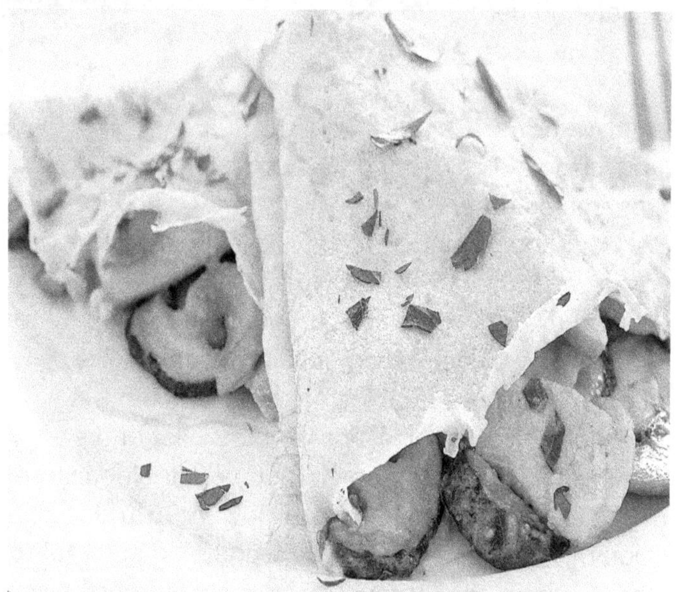

Ingredients:
- 1 lb boneless, skinless chicken breast, cooked and shredded
- 1 cup mixed mushrooms (button, cremini, shiitake), sautéed
- 1 cup spinach leaves
- 1/2 cup grated Parmesan cheese
- 1/4 cup low-carb crepe batter (check the carb count)
- 1 egg, beaten
- 1 tsp vanilla extract
- Salt and pepper, to taste

Instructions:
1. In a bowl, mix together chicken, mushrooms, spinach, and Parmesan cheese.
2. In a separate bowl, whisk together crepe batter, egg, and vanilla extract.
3. Heat a small non-stick pan over medium heat. Pour in the crepe batter and cook until the bottom is light brown.
4. Flip the crepe and fill with the chicken-mushroom mixture. Roll up and serve hot.

Note: You can adjust the filling to your liking and add other low-carb ingredients like diced bell peppers or zucchini. Also, make sure to check the carb count on the crepe batter to ensure it fits within your daily carb limit.

7. Korean-Style Chicken And Vegetable Skewers

Ingredients:
- 1 lb boneless, skinless chicken breast, cut into bite-sized pieces
- 1 cup mixed vegetables (bell peppers, zucchini, onions, mushrooms)
- 1/4 cup Gochujang (Korean chili paste)
- 2 tbsp soy sauce
- 2 tbsp brown sugar
- 2 tbsp garlic, minced
- 1 tsp ginger, grated
- 1/4 cup chopped green onions, for garnish

- 1/4 cup toasted sesame seeds, for garnish

Instructions:
1. Preheat the grill to medium-high heat.
2. In a large bowl, whisk together Gochujang, soy sauce, brown sugar, garlic, and ginger.
3. Add the chicken and vegetables to the bowl and toss to coat.
4. Thread the chicken and vegetables onto skewers.
5. Grill for 10-12 minutes, or until the chicken is cooked through.
6. Garnish with green onions and sesame seeds. Serve hot.

Note: You can adjust the level of spiciness to your liking by adding more or less Gochujang. Also, make sure to choose low-carb vegetables like bell peppers and zucchini to keep the dish low in carbs.

8. Chicken And Spinach Stuffed Portobellos

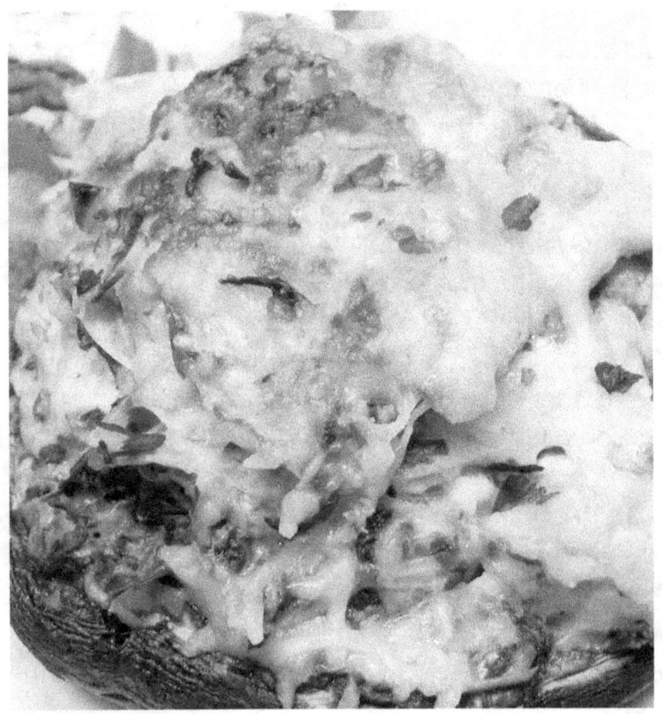

Ingredients:

- 4 large Portobello mushrooms, stems removed and caps cleaned
- 1 lb boneless, skinless chicken breast, cooked and shredded
- 1 cup fresh spinach leaves
- 1/2 cup grated Parmesan cheese
- 1/4 cup low-carb breadcrumbs (check the carb count)
- 2 cloves garlic, minced

- 1 tsp dried thyme
- Salt and pepper, to taste
- 2 tbsp olive oil

Instructions:
1. Preheat the oven to 375°F (190°C).
2. In a bowl, mix together chicken, spinach, Parmesan cheese, breadcrumbs, garlic, and thyme.
3. Stuff each mushroom cap with the chicken mixture, dividing it evenly.
4. Drizzle the tops with olive oil and season with salt and pepper.
5. Bake for 15-20 minutes, or until the mushrooms are tender and the filling is heated through.
6. Serve hot and enjoy!

Note: Adjust the filling to your liking and add other low-carb ingredients like diced bell peppers or zucchini. Also, make sure to check the carb count on the breadcrumbs to ensure they fit within your daily carb limit.

9. Turkey And Cranberry Meatloaf

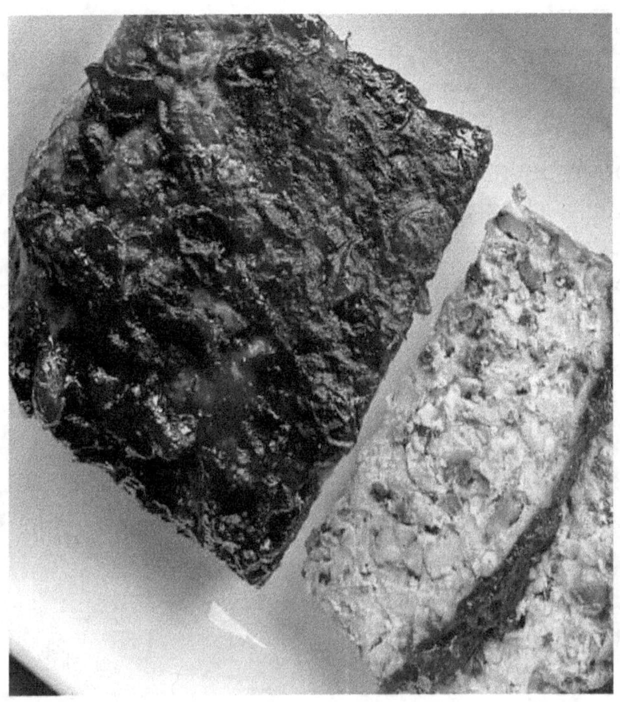

Ingredients:
- 1 lb ground turkey
- 1/2 cup almond flour
- 1/4 cup grated cheddar cheese
- 1/4 cup dried cranberries
- 1/4 cup chopped pecans
- 2 cloves garlic, minced
- 1 tsp salt
- 1/2 tsp black pepper
- 1/4 tsp paprika
- 1/4 tsp cayenne pepper (optional)

- 1 egg, beaten
- 1/4 cup low-carb ketchup (check the carb count)

Instructions:
1. Preheat the oven to 375°F (190°C).
2. In a large bowl, combine ground turkey, almond flour, cheese, cranberries, pecans, garlic, salt, pepper, paprika, and cayenne pepper (if using).
3. Mix well with your hands or a wooden spoon until just combined.
4. Add the beaten egg and mix until the meat is just holding together.
5. Shape into a loaf and place on a baking sheet lined with parchment paper.
6. Brush the top with low-carb ketchup.
7. Bake for 45-50 minutes, or until the meatloaf is cooked through and the internal temperature reaches 165°F (74°C).
8. Let rest for 10 minutes before slicing and serving.

Note: You can adjust the amount of cranberries and pecans to your liking, and also add other low-carb ingredients like diced onions or bell peppers. Make sure to check the carb count on the ketchup to ensure it fits within your daily carb limit.

10. Turkish-Style Stuffed Bell Peppers

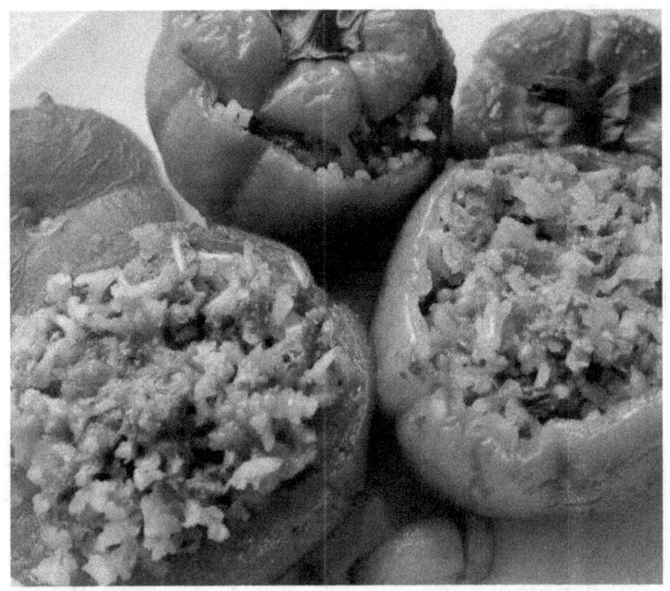

Ingredients:
- 4 large bell peppers, any color
- 1 lb ground turkey
- 1 cup cooked cauliflower rice
- 1/2 cup chopped fresh parsley
- 1/4 cup crumbled feta cheese
- 1/4 cup chopped fresh mint
- 2 cloves garlic, minced
- 1 tsp ground cumin
- 1 tsp paprika
- Salt and pepper, to taste
- 2 tbsp olive oil

Instructions:
1. Preheat the oven to 375°F (190°C).
2. Cut the tops off the bell peppers and remove the seeds and membranes.
3. In a bowl, mix together ground turkey, cauliflower rice, parsley, feta cheese, mint, garlic, cumin, paprika, salt, and pepper.
4. Stuff each bell pepper with the turkey mixture, dividing it evenly.
5. Drizzle the tops with olive oil and cover with the bell pepper tops.
6. Bake for 30-35 minutes, or until the bell peppers are tender and the filling is cooked through.
7. Serve hot and enjoy!

Note: You can adjust the filling to your liking and add other low-carb ingredients like diced onions or zucchini. Also, make sure to check the carb count on the ingredients to ensure they fit within your daily carb limit.

11. Garlic Shrimp

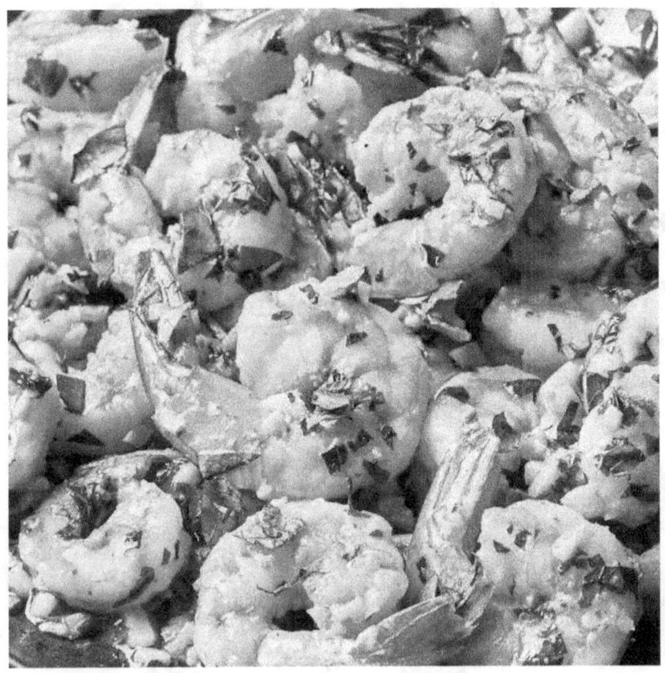

Ingredients:
- 1 pound large shrimp, peeled and deveined
- 4 cloves garlic, minced
- 1/4 cup olive oil
- 1/2 teaspoon salt
- 1/4 teaspoon black pepper
- 1/4 teaspoon red pepper flakes (optional)
- 1/4 cup chopped fresh parsley
- 1/4 cup grated Parmesan cheese (optional)

Instructions:
1. In a large skillet, heat olive oil over medium-high heat.

2. Add garlic and sauté for 1-2 minutes until fragrant.
3. Add shrimp and sauté for 2-3 minutes per side until pink and cooked through.
4. Season with salt, pepper, and red pepper flakes (if using).
5. Stir in parsley and Parmesan cheese (if using).
6. Serve hot and enjoy!

Note: You can adjust the amount of garlic and red pepper flakes to your liking. Also, make sure to check the carb count on the Parmesan cheese to ensure it fits within your daily carb limit.

12. Baked Salmon With Lemon And Herbs

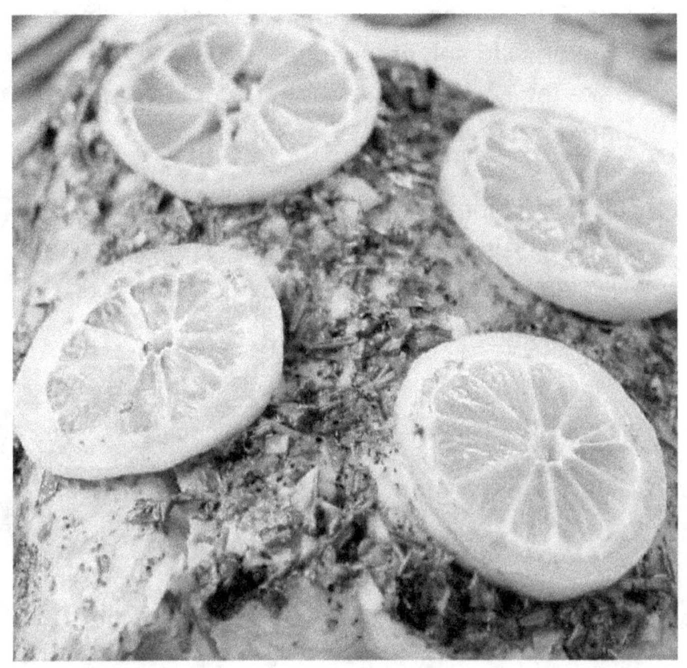

Ingredients:
- 4 salmon filets (6 oz each)
- 2 lemons, sliced
- 1/4 cup olive oil
- 4 tbsp chopped fresh rosemary
- 4 tbsp chopped fresh thyme
- Salt and pepper, to taste

Instructions:
1. Preheat the oven to 400°F (200°C).
2. Line a baking sheet with parchment paper.

3. Place salmon filets on the baking sheet.
4. Drizzle olive oil over the salmon.
5. Place a slice of lemon on top of each filet.
6. Sprinkle rosemary and thyme over the salmon.
7. Season with salt and pepper to taste.
8. Bake for 12-15 minutes or until cooked through.
9. Serve hot and enjoy!

Note: Adjust the amount of herbs and lemon to your liking. Also, make sure to check the carb count on the ingredients to ensure they fit within your daily carb limit.

13. Tuna Steak With Lemon And Herb

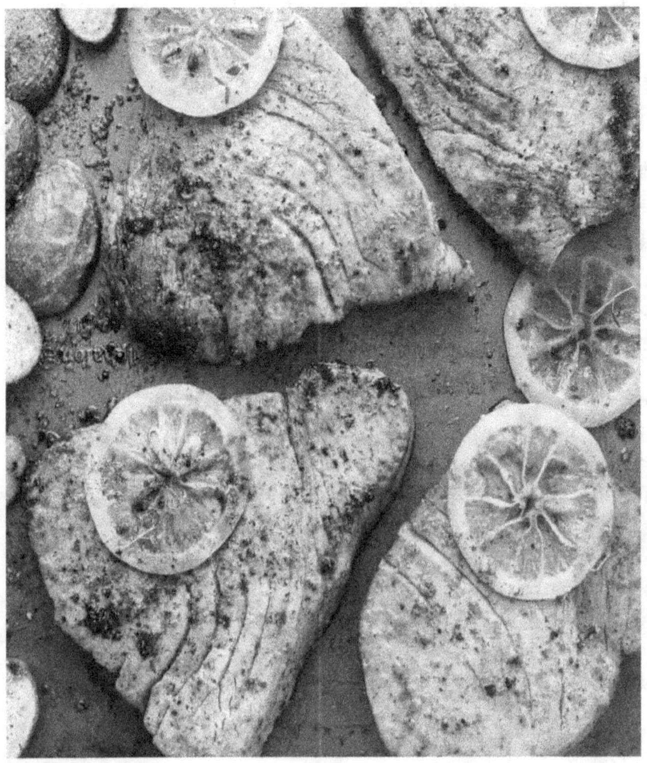

Ingredients:
- 4 tuna steaks (6 oz each)
- 1/4 cup freshly squeezed lemon juice
- 2 tbsp olive oil
- 4 tbsp chopped fresh rosemary
- 4 tbsp chopped fresh thyme
- Salt and pepper, to taste

Instructions:

1. Preheat the grill or grill pan to medium-high heat.
2. In a small bowl, whisk together lemon juice, olive oil, rosemary, thyme, salt, and pepper.
3. Brush the mixture evenly onto both sides of the tuna steaks.
4. Grill for 4-5 minutes per side, or until cooked to your desired level of doneness.
5. Serve hot and enjoy!

Note: You can adjust the amount of lemon juice and herbs to your liking. Also, make sure to check the carb count on the tuna steaks to ensure they fit within your daily carb limit. Some tuna steaks may contain added ingredients that increase the carb count.

14. Lobster And Avocado Salad

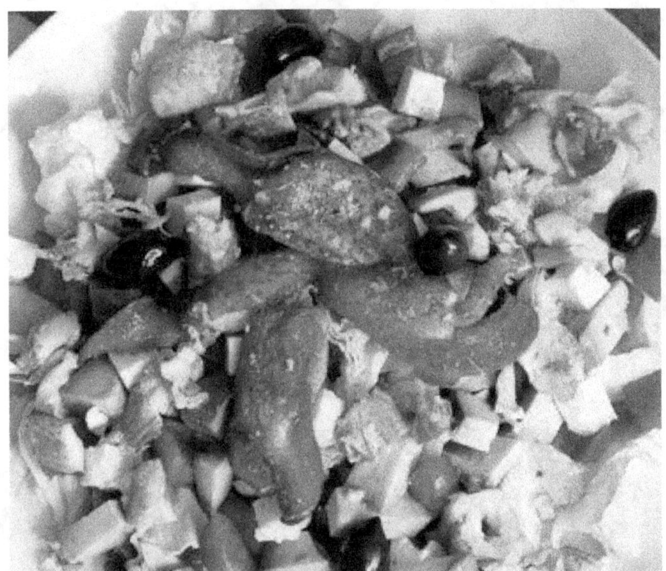

Ingredients:
- 1 pound cooked lobster meat, diced
- 2 ripe avocados, diced
- 1/2 cup chopped red onion
- 1/4 cup chopped fresh cilantro
- 2 tablespoons freshly squeezed lime juice
- Salt and pepper, to taste

Instructions:
1. In a large bowl, combine lobster meat, avocado, red onion, and cilantro.
2. Squeeze lime juice over the top and toss gently to combine.
3. Season with salt and pepper to taste.
4. Serve immediately and enjoy!

Note: You can adjust the amount of lime juice and cilantro to your liking. Also, make sure to check the carb count on the lobster meat to ensure it fits within your daily carb limit. Some lobster meat may contain added ingredients that increase the carb count.

15. Grilled Scallops With Garlic Butter

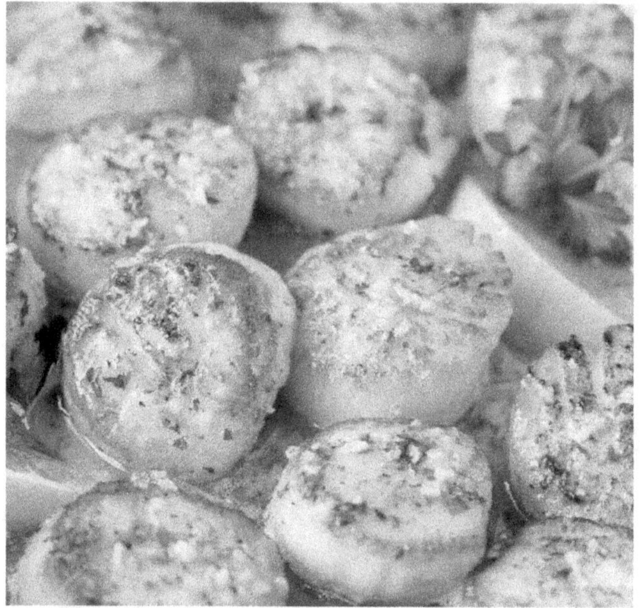

Ingredients:
- 12 large scallops
- 4 cloves garlic, minced
- 2 tablespoons unsalted butter, softened

- 2 tablespoons freshly squeezed lemon juice
- Salt and pepper, to taste
- Fresh parsley, chopped (optional)

Instructions:
1. Preheat the grill to medium-high heat.
2. In a small bowl, mix together garlic, butter, lemon juice, salt, and pepper.
3. Brush the mixture evenly onto both sides of the scallops.
4. Grill for 2-3 minutes per side, or until cooked through.
5. Garnish with chopped parsley, if desired.
6. Serve hot and enjoy!

Note: You can adjust the amount of garlic and lemon juice to your liking. Also, make sure to check the carb count on the scallops to ensure they fit within your daily carb limit. Some scallops may contain added ingredients that increase the carb count.

Chapter Four

Sides And Vegetables

1. Cauliflower Rice And Vegetable Stir-Fry With Broccoli And Bell Peppers

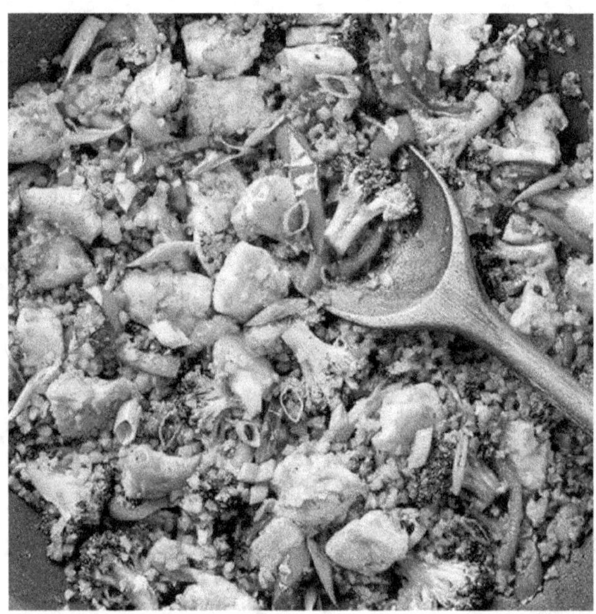

Ingredients:
- 1 head of cauliflower
- 2 cups broccoli florets
- 1 cup sliced bell peppers
- 2 tablespoons olive oil

- 1 clove garlic, minced
- Salt and pepper, to taste
- Optional: 1/4 cup grated Parmesan cheese

Instructions:
1. Pulse cauliflower in a food processor until it resembles rice.
2. Heat olive oil in a large skillet over medium heat.
3. Add garlic and sauté for 1 minute.
4. Add broccoli and bell peppers and cook until tender-crisp.
5. Add the cauliflower "rice" and stir-fry until combined with the vegetables.
6. Season with salt, pepper, and Parmesan cheese (if using).
7. Serve hot and enjoy!

This recipe combines the Cauliflower Rice grain recipe with the Broccoli and Bell Peppers veggie recipes. You can adjust the ingredients and seasonings to your liking, and also add other veggies or protein sources to make it a complete meal. Remember to check the carb count and adjust the serving size accordingly.

2. Zucchini Noodles With Tomato And Mushroom Sauce

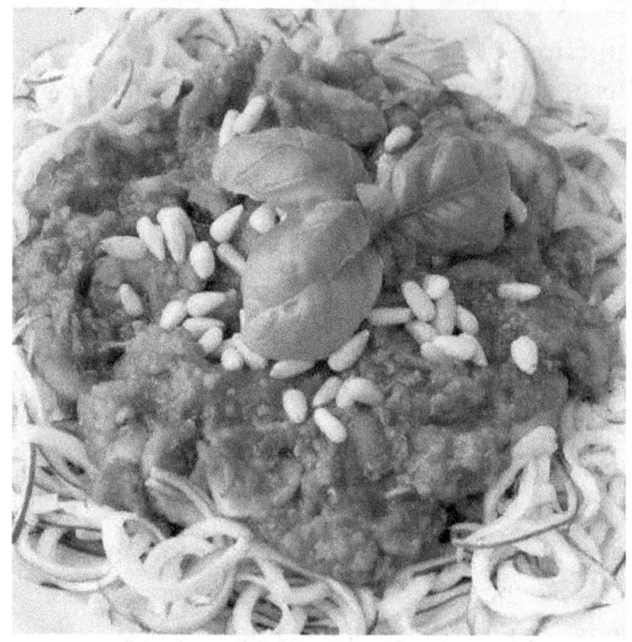

Ingredients:

- 2 medium zucchinis
- 1 cup sliced mushrooms
- 1 cup diced tomatoes
- 2 cloves garlic, minced
- 1/4 cup olive oil
- Salt and pepper, to taste
- Optional: 1/4 cup grated Parmesan cheese

Instructions:

1. Spiralize a zucchini into noodles.
2. Heat olive oil in a large skillet over medium heat.

3. Add garlic and sauté for 1 minute.
4. Add mushrooms and cook until tender.
5. Add diced tomatoes and cook until the sauce thickens.
6. Add the zucchini noodles and toss with the tomato-mushroom sauce.
7. Season with salt, pepper, and Parmesan cheese (if using).
8. Serve hot and enjoy!

You can adjust the ingredients and seasonings to your liking, and also add other protein sources or veggies to make it a complete meal. Remember to check the carb count and adjust the serving size accordingly.

3. Avocado Toast On Almond Flour Bread With Roasted Brussels Sprouts

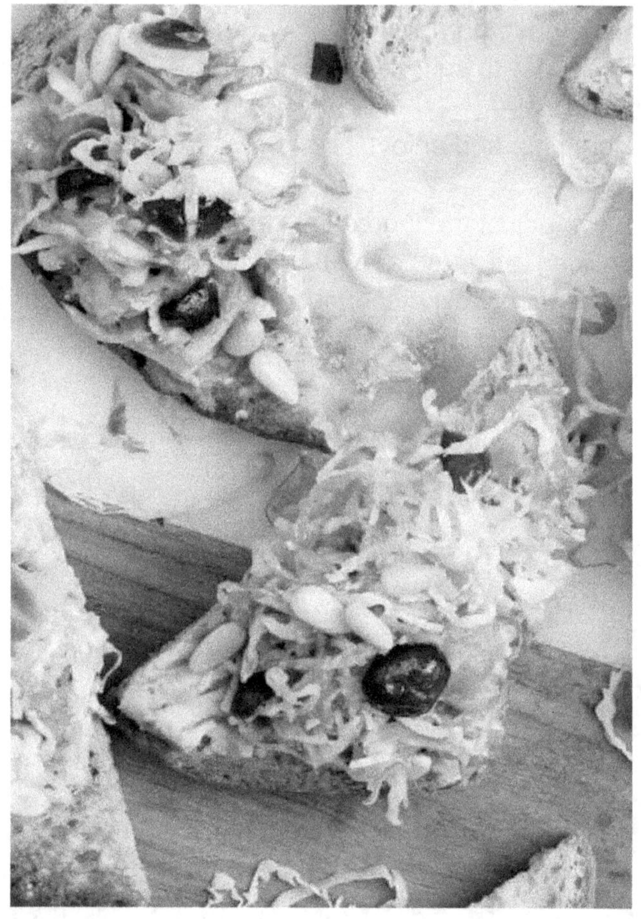

Ingredients:
- 1 loaf Almond Flour Bread
- 2 ripe avocados, mashed

- 1 pound Brussels sprouts, trimmed and halved
- 2 tablespoons olive oil
- Salt and pepper, to taste
- Optional: 1/4 cup cherry tomatoes, halved

Instructions:
1. Preheat the oven to 400°F (200°C).
2. Slice the Almond Flour Bread into toast.
3. Spread mashed avocado on each slice.
4. Toss Brussels sprouts with olive oil, salt, and pepper, and roast in the oven until tender.
5. Top the avocado toast with roasted Brussels sprouts and cherry tomatoes (if using).
6. Serve and enjoy!

4. Cauliflower And Mushroom Tacos With Coconut Flour Tortillas

Ingredients:
- 4 Coconut Flour Tortillas
- 1 head of cauliflower, grated
- 1 cup sliced mushrooms
- 2 cloves garlic, minced
- 1/4 cup olive oil
- Salt and pepper, to taste
- Optional: 1/4 cup sliced avocado, 1/4 cup sour cream

Instructions:
1. Heat olive oil in a large skillet over medium heat.

2. Add garlic and sauté for 1 minute.
3. Add mushrooms and cook until tender.
4. Add grated cauliflower and cook until tender.
5. Warm Coconut Flour Tortillas according to package instructions.
6. Fill tortillas with cauliflower-mushroom mixture and top with avocado and sour cream (if using).
7. Serve and enjoy!

5. Cauliflower and Broccoli Cheese Bites On Flaxseed Meal Crackers

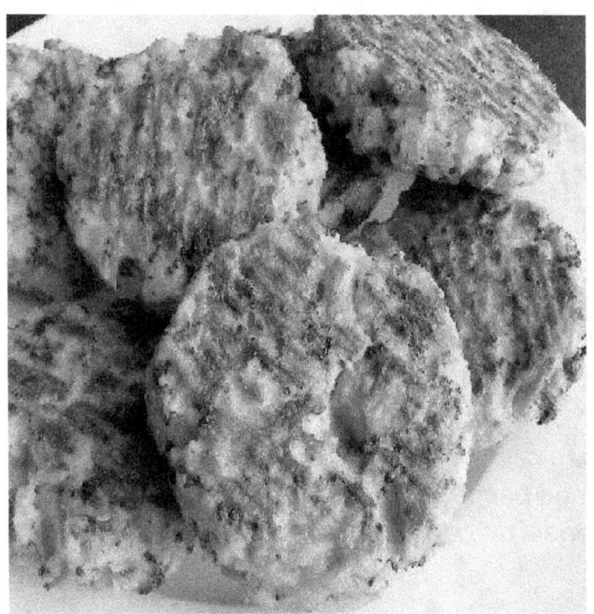

Ingredients:
- 1 cup Flaxseed Meal Crackers

- 1 head of cauliflower, grated
- 2 cups broccoli florets
- 1 cup shredded cheese
- 1/4 cup almond flour
- 1 egg, beaten
- Salt and pepper, to taste

Instructions:
1. Preheat the oven to 375°F (190°C).
2. Mix grated cauliflower, broccoli florets, shredded cheese, almond flour, and beaten egg in a bowl.
3. Spoon the mixture onto Flaxseed Meal Crackers.
4. Bake in the oven until the cheese is melted and the crackers are crispy.
5. Serve and enjoy!

6. Avocado And Asparagus Bites On Flaxseed Meal Crackers

Ingredients:
- 1 cup Flaxseed Meal Crackers
- 2 ripe avocados, mashed
- 1 pound fresh asparagus, trimmed
- 1/4 cup cherry tomatoes, halved
- Salt and pepper, to taste
- Optional: 1/4 cup crumbled feta cheese

Instructions:
1. Preheat the oven to 375°F (190°C).
2. Toss asparagus with olive oil, salt, and pepper, and roast in the oven until tender.

3. Spread mashed avocado on Flaxseed Meal Crackers.
4. Top with roasted asparagus, cherry tomatoes, and feta cheese (if using).
5. Serve and enjoy!

7. Cauliflower And Mushroom Cauliflower Rice Bowl With Coconut Flour Crackers

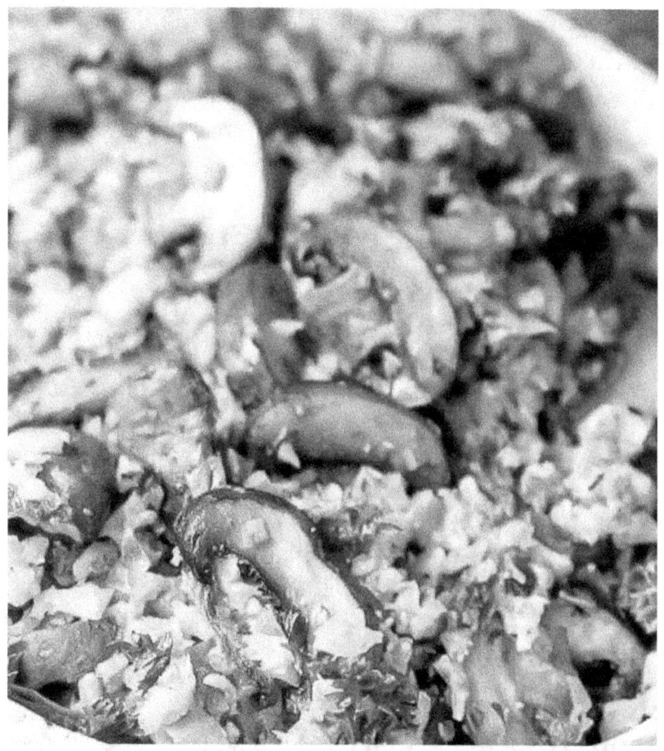

Ingredients:

- 1 head of cauliflower
- 1 cup cauliflower rice
- 1 cup sliced mushrooms
- 2 cloves garlic, minced
- 1/4 cup coconut oil
- Salt and pepper, to taste
- 4 Coconut Flour Crackers

Instructions:
1. Pulse cauliflower in a food processor until it resembles rice.
2. Heat coconut oil in a large skillet over medium heat.
3. Add garlic and sauté for 1 minute.
4. Add mushrooms and cook until tender.
5. Add cauliflower rice and cook until combined with the mushroom mixture.
6. Serve in a bowl with Coconut Flour Crackers on the side.

8. Zucchini Noodles With Broccoli And Almond Flour Breadsticks

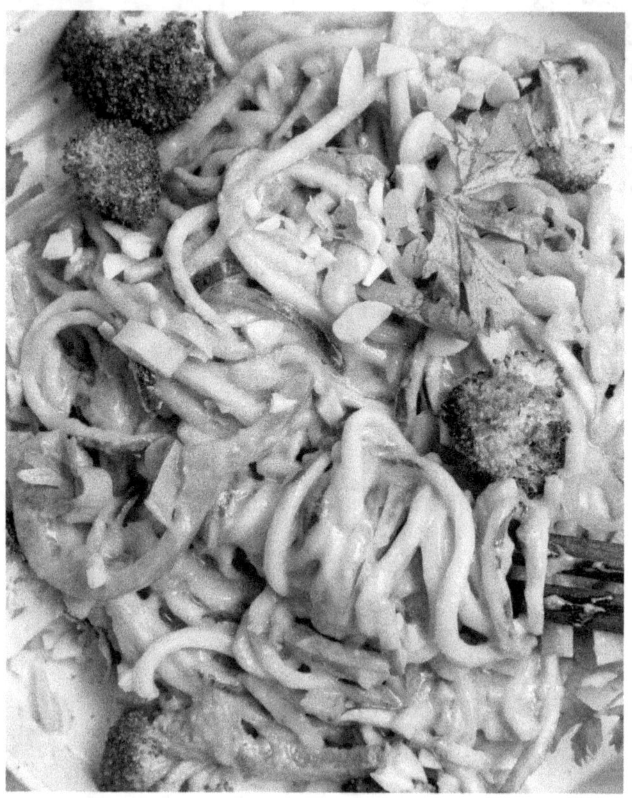

Ingredients:
- 2 medium zucchinis
- 2 cups broccoli florets
- 1/4 cup almond flour
- 1/4 cup grated Parmesan cheese
- 1 egg, beaten
- Salt and pepper, to taste

- 4 Almond Flour Breadsticks

Instructions:
1. Spiralize a zucchini into noodles.
2. Steam broccoli until tender.
3. Mix almond flour, Parmesan cheese, and beaten egg in a bowl.
4. Add the mixture to the zucchini noodles and toss to combine.
5. Serve with steamed broccoli and Almond Flour Breadsticks on the side.

9. Cauliflower Rice And Asparagus With Coconut Flour Tortilla

Ingredients:
- 1 head of cauliflower
- 1 pound fresh asparagus, trimmed
- 1/4 cup coconut oil
- Salt and pepper, to taste
- 1 Coconut Flour Tortilla

Instructions:
1. Pulse cauliflower in a food processor until it resembles rice.
2. Heat coconut oil in a large skillet over medium heat.
3. Add asparagus and cook until tender.
4. Add cauliflower rice and cook until combined with the asparagus.

5. Serve in a Coconut Flour Tortilla for a low-carb wrap.

10. Flaxseed Meal Crackers With Avocado And Bell Peppers

Ingredients:
- 1 cup Flaxseed Meal Crackers
- 2 ripe avocados, mashed
- 2 bell peppers, sliced
- Salt and pepper, to taste

Instructions:
1. Spread mashed avocado on Flaxseed Meal Crackers.
2. Top with sliced bell peppers.
3. Serve and enjoy!

Desserts

1. Keto Cheesecake

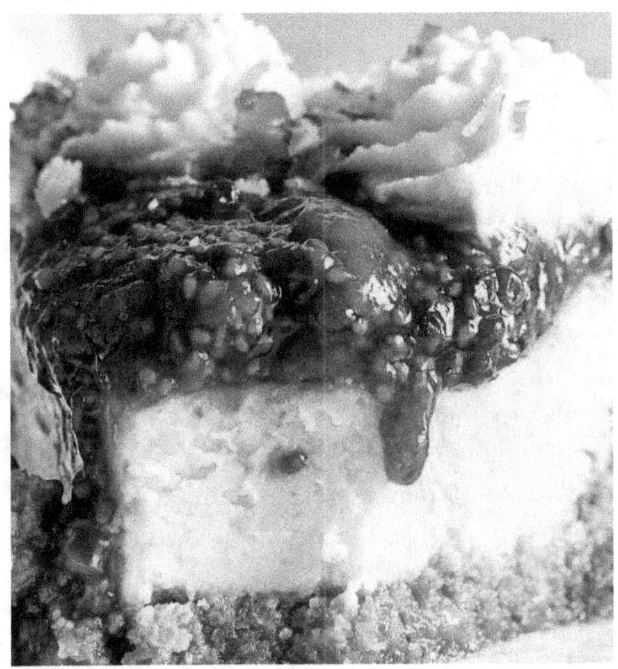

Ingredients:
- Crust:
    - 1 1/2 cups almond flour
    - 1/4 cup granulated sweetener (e.g., Swerve or Erythritol)
    - 1/4 cup melted butter
- Filling:
    - 16 ounces cream cheese, softened
    - 1/2 cup granulated sweetener (e.g., Swerve or Erythritol)

  - 4 large eggs, separated
  - 1 teaspoon vanilla extract
- Topping:
  - 1 cup sour cream
  - 1/2 cup granulated sweetener (e.g., Swerve or Erythritol)
  - 1/2 teaspoon vanilla extract

Instructions:
1. Preheat the oven to 325°F (165°C).
2. Prepare the crust: Mix almond flour, sweetener, and melted butter in a bowl. Press into a lined or greased 8-inch square baking dish.
3. Prepare the filling: Beat cream cheese until smooth. Add sweetener, egg yolks (one at a time), and vanilla extract. Mix well.
4. Pour filling over the crust.
5. Bake for 25-30 minutes or until edges are set.
6. Prepare topping: Mix sour cream, sweetener, and vanilla extract.
7. Top cheesecake with sour cream mixture.
8. Refrigerate for at least 4 hours or overnight.
9. Cut into slices and serve!

Note: Net carbs per slice (1/12 of the recipe): 5g

2. Keto Coconut Cream Pie

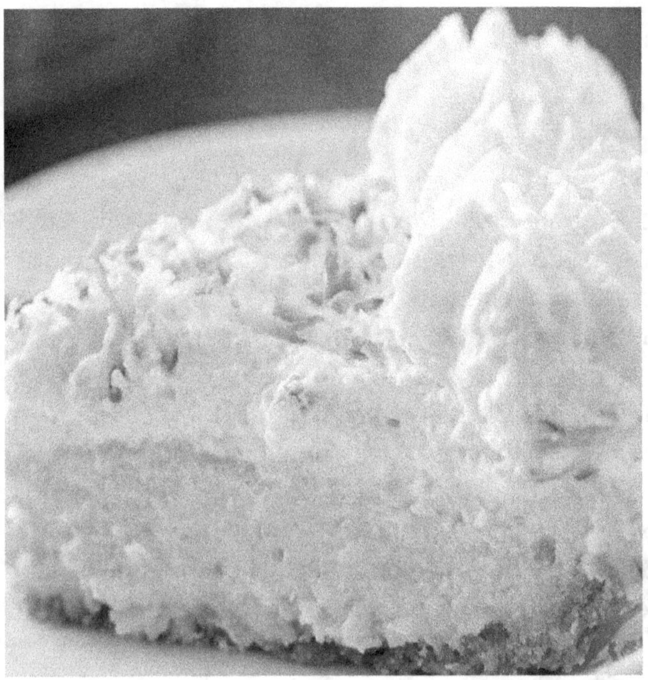

Ingredients:
- Crust:
    - 1 1/2 cups almond flour
    - 1/4 cup granulated sweetener (e.g., Swerve or Erythritol)
    - 1/4 cup melted coconut oil
- Filling:
    - 1 can (14 oz) full-fat coconut milk
    - 1/2 cup granulated sweetener (e.g., Swerve or Erythritol)
    - 3 large egg yolks
    - 1 teaspoon vanilla extract

- Whipped Cream:
    - 1 can (14 oz) full-fat coconut milk, chilled
    - 2 tablespoons granulated sweetener (e.g.,
Swerve or Erythritol)

Instructions:
1. Preheat the oven to 350°F (180°C).
2. Prepare crust: Mix almond flour, sweetener, and melted coconut oil in a bowl. Press into a lined or greased 9-inch pie dish.
3. Bake crust for 12-15 minutes or until lightly golden.
4. Prepare filling: Mix coconut milk, sweetener, egg yolks, and vanilla extract in a bowl. Pour into the baked crust.
5. Bake for 15-18 minutes or until filling is set.
6. Prepare whipped cream: Chill coconut milk in the refrigerator overnight. Open the can and scoop out solid coconut cream. Mix with sweetener and vanilla extract.
7. Top pie with whipped cream and refrigerate for at least 2 hours before serving.

Note: Net carbs per serving (1/8 of the recipe): 5g

3. Keto Pecan Pie

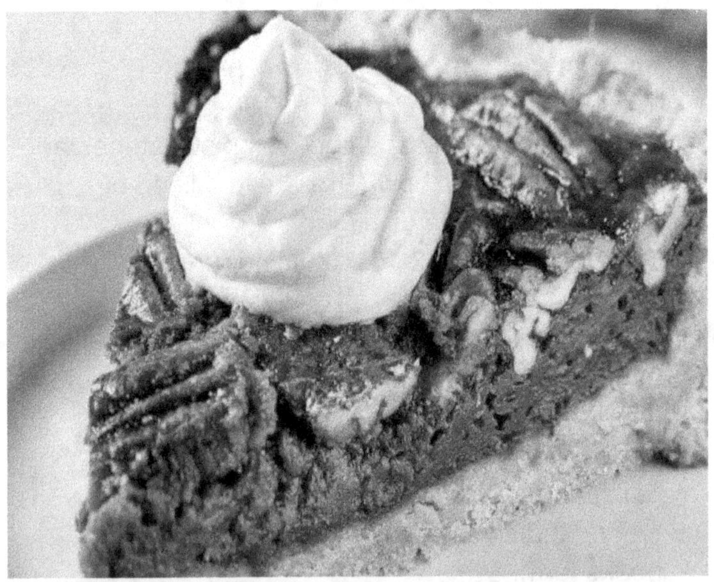

Ingredients:
- Crust:
    - 1 1/2 cups almond flour
    - 1/4 cup granulated sweetener (e.g., Swerve or Erythritol)
    - 1/4 cup melted butter
- Filling:
    - 1 cup pecan halves
    - 1/2 cup granulated sweetener (e.g., Swerve or Erythritol)
    - 1/4 cup melted butter
    - 2 large eggs
    - 1 teaspoon vanilla extract
- Whipped Cream (optional):
    - 1 cup heavy cream

- 2 tablespoons granulated sweetener (e.g., Swerve or Erythritol)

Instructions:
1. Preheat the oven to 350°F (180°C).
2. Prepare crust: Mix almond flour, sweetener, and melted butter in a bowl. Press into a lined or greased 9-inch pie dish.
3. Bake crust for 12-15 minutes or until lightly golden.
4. Prepare filling: Mix pecans, sweetener, melted butter, eggs, and vanilla extract in a bowl. Pour into the baked crust.
5. Bake for 25-30 minutes or until filling is set.
6. Prepare whipped cream (if using): Mix heavy cream and sweetener in a bowl. Whip until stiff peaks form.
7. Top pie with whipped cream (if using) and refrigerate for at least 2 hours before serving.

Note: Net carbs per serving (1/8 of the recipe): 5g

4. Keto Chocolate Silk Pie

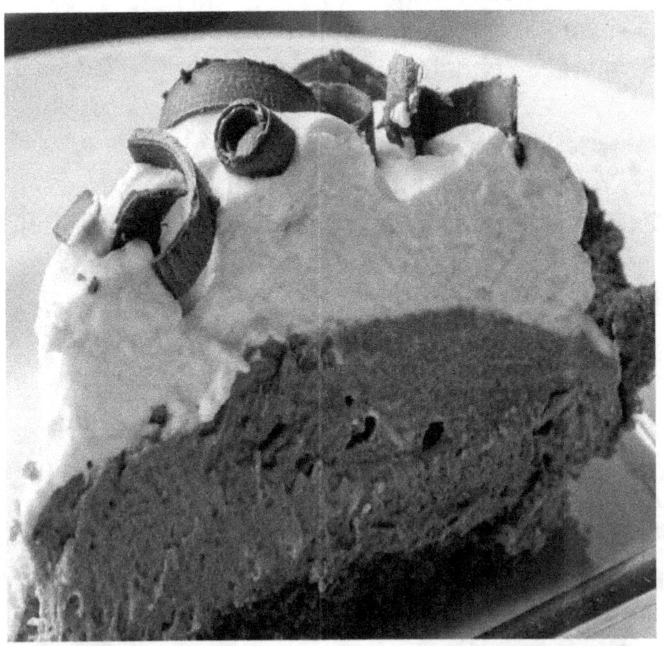

Ingredients:
- Crust:
    - 1 1/2 cups almond flour
    - 1/4 cup granulated sweetener (e.g., Swerve or Erythritol)
    - 1/4 cup melted coconut oil
- Filling:
    - 8 ounces cream cheese, softened
    - 1/2 cup granulated sweetener (e.g., Swerve or Erythritol)
    - 2 large eggs
    - 1/2 cup unsweetened cocoa powder
    - 1 teaspoon vanilla extract

- Whipped Cream (optional):
    - 1 cup heavy cream
    - 2 tablespoons granulated sweetener (e.g.,
Swerve or Erythritol)

Instructions:
1. Preheat the oven to 350°F (180°C).
2. Prepare crust: Mix almond flour, sweetener, and melted coconut oil in a bowl. Press into a lined or greased 9-inch pie dish.
3. Bake crust for 12-15 minutes or until lightly golden.
4. Prepare filling: Mix cream cheese, sweetener, eggs, cocoa powder, and vanilla extract in a bowl. Pour into the baked crust.
5. Bake for 25-30 minutes or until filling is set.
6. Prepare whipped cream (if using): Mix heavy cream and sweetener in a bowl. Whip until stiff peaks form.
7. Top pie with whipped cream (if using) and refrigerate for at least 2 hours before serving.

Note: Net carbs per serving (1/8 of the recipe): 5g

5. Keto Cheesecake With Almond Flour Crust

Ingredients:
- Crust:
    - 2 cups almond flour

- 1/4 cup granulated sweetener (e.g., Swerve or Erythritol)
    - 1/4 cup melted butter
- Filling:
    - 16 ounces cream cheese, softened
    - 1/2 cup granulated sweetener (e.g., Swerve or Erythritol)
    - 4 large eggs, separated
    - 1 teaspoon vanilla extract
- Topping (optional):
    - 1 cup sour cream
    - 1/2 cup granulated sweetener (e.g., Swerve or Erythritol)
    - 1/2 teaspoon vanilla extract

Instructions:
1. Preheat the oven to 325°F (165°C).
2. Prepare crust: Mix almond flour, sweetener, and melted butter in a bowl. Press into a lined or greased 9-inch springform pan.
3. Bake the crust for 15-20 minutes or until lightly golden.
4. Prepare filling: Beat cream cheese until smooth. Add sweetener, egg yolks (one at a time), and vanilla extract. Mix well.
5. Pour filling over the crust.
6. Bake for 45-50 minutes or until edges are set.
7. Prepare topping (if using): Mix sour cream, sweetener, and vanilla extract.
8. Top cheesecake with sour cream mixture (if using) and refrigerate for at least 4 hours or overnight.

Note: Net carbs per serving (1/12 of the recipe): 5g

6. Low Carb Cookie Dough Ice Cream

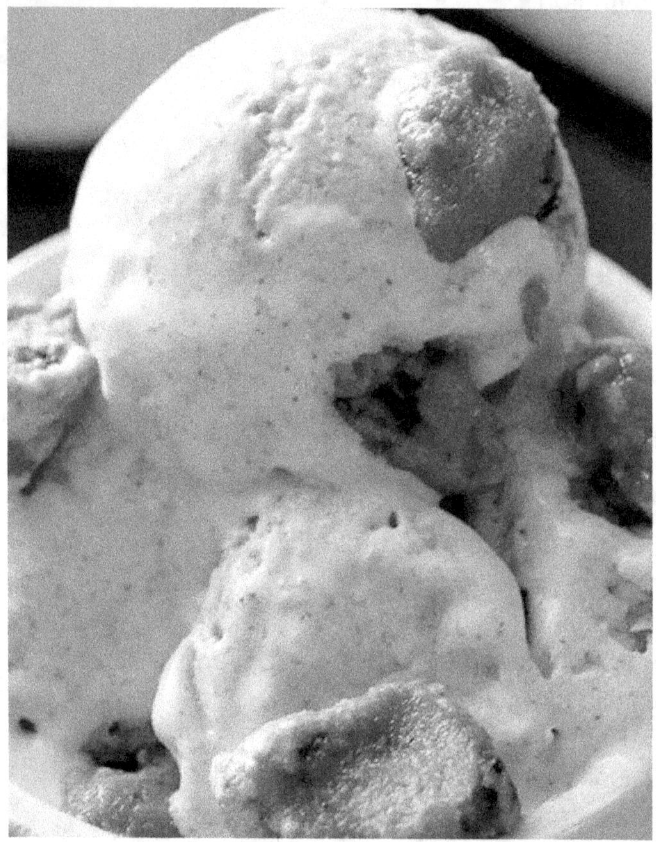

Ingredients:
- 2 cups heavy cream
- 1/2 cup unsalted butter, softened

- 1/2 cup granulated sweetener (e.g., Swerve or Erythritol)
- 2 large eggs
- 1 teaspoon vanilla extract
- 1 cup low-carb cookie dough chunks (made with almond flour and sweetener)

Instructions:
1. In a large mixing bowl, combine heavy cream, butter, sweetener, eggs, and vanilla extract. Mix until smooth.
2. Add low-carb cookie dough chunks and mix until well combined.
3. Pour mixture into an ice cream maker and churn according to manufacturer's instructions.
4. Freeze for at least 2 hours before serving.

Note: If you don't have an ice cream maker, you can also freeze the mixture in a shallow metal pan and blend it in a food processor once it's frozen solid.

Macro breakdown per serving (1/2 cup):

- Calories: 320
- Protein: 6g
- Fat: 28g
- Carbohydrates: 5g
- Fiber: 1g
- Net Carbs: 4g

7. Keto Vanilla Ice Cream

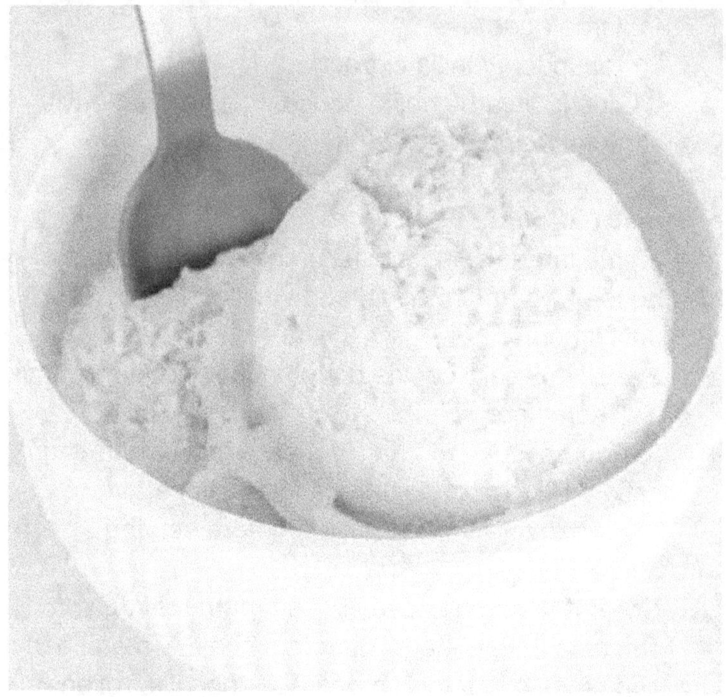

Ingredients:
- 2 cups heavy cream
- 1/2 cup unsalted butter, softened
- 1/2 cup granulated sweetener (e.g., Swerve or Erythritol)
- 2 large eggs
- 1 teaspoon vanilla extract

Instructions:
1. In a large mixing bowl, combine heavy cream, butter, sweetener, eggs, and vanilla extract. Mix until smooth.

2. Pour mixture into an ice cream maker and churn according to manufacturer's instructions.
3. Freeze for at least 2 hours before serving.

Note: If you don't have an ice cream maker, you can also freeze the mixture in a shallow metal pan and blend it in a food processor once it's frozen solid.

Macro breakdown per serving (1/2 cup):

- Calories: 350
- Protein: 6g
- Fat: 32g
- Carbohydrates: 5g
- Fiber: 1g
- Net Carbs: 4g

Make sure to choose a sweetener that is suitable for a keto diet and adjust the amount to your taste. Also, keep in mind that the macro breakdown may vary depending on the specific ingredients and portion sizes used.

8. Mason Jar Ice Cream

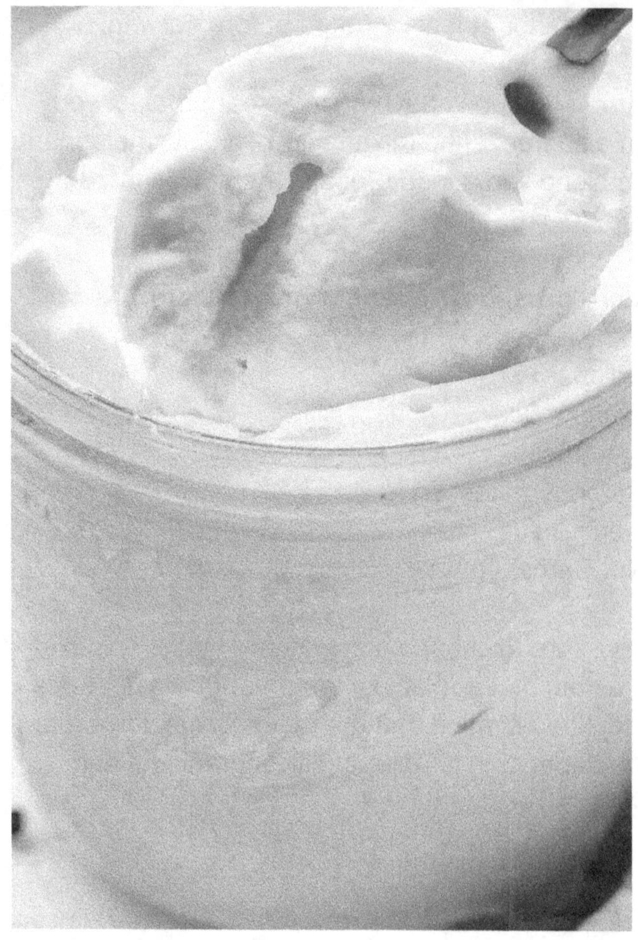

Ingredients:
- 1 pint heavy cream
- 1/2 cup unsalted butter, softened
- 1/2 cup granulated sweetener (e.g., Swerve or Erythritol)
- 2 large eggs

- 1 teaspoon vanilla extract

Instructions:
1. In a large mixing bowl, combine heavy cream, butter, sweetener, eggs, and vanilla extract. Mix until smooth.
2. Pour mixture into 4-6 mason jars, leaving about 1 inch of space at the top.
3. Place jars in the freezer and every 30 minutes, remove and blend the mixture with an immersion blender until smooth and creamy.
4. Repeat the process for 2-3 hours, or until desired consistency is reached.

Macro breakdown per serving (1 jar):

- Calories: 320
- Protein: 6g
- Fat: 28g
- Carbohydrates: 5g
- Fiber: 1g
- Net Carbs: 4g

9. Dairy-Free Keto Vanilla Ice Cream

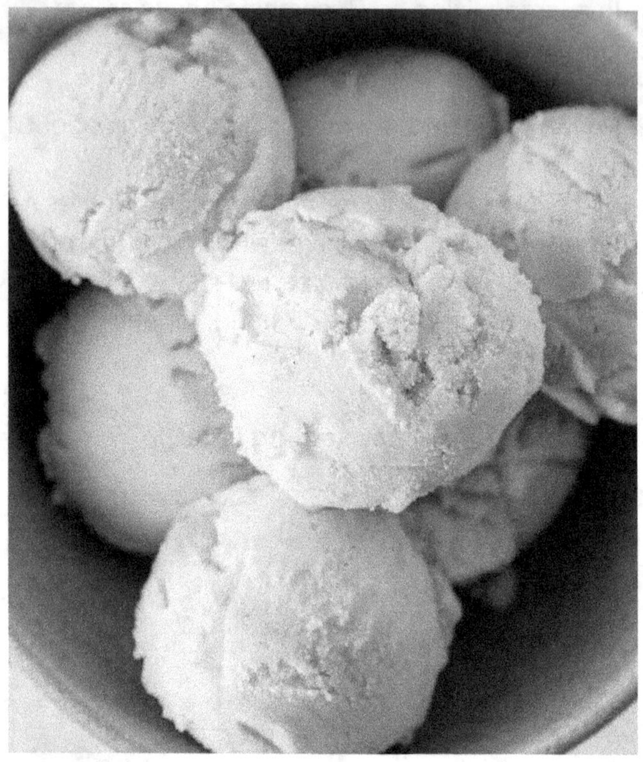

Ingredients:
- 1 1/2 cups full-fat coconut milk
- 1/4 cup unsweetened almond milk
- 1/4 cup granulated sweetener (e.g., Swerve or Erythritol)
- 1/4 cup melted coconut oil
- 2 large eggs
- 1 teaspoon vanilla extract

Instructions:
1. In a blender, combine coconut milk, almond milk, sweetener, melted coconut oil, eggs, and vanilla extract. Blend until smooth.
2. Pour mixture into an ice cream maker and churn according to manufacturer's instructions.
3. Freeze for at least 2 hours before serving.

Note: If you don't have an ice cream maker, you can also freeze the mixture in a shallow metal pan and blend it in a food processor once it's frozen solid.

Macro breakdown per serving (1/2 cup):

- Calories: 320
- Protein: 6g
- Fat: 28g
- Carbohydrates: 5g
- Fiber: 1g
- Net Carbs: 4g

10. 3-Ingredient Keto Ice Cream

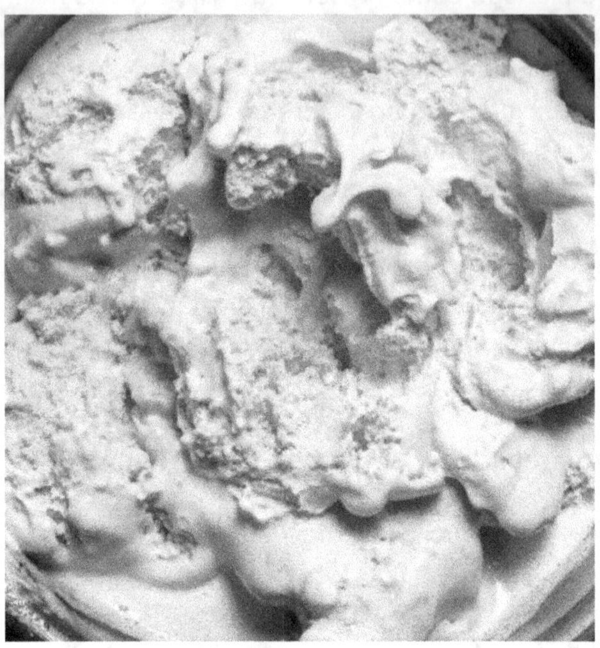

Ingredients:
- 1 1/2 cups frozen berries (such as blueberries, strawberries, or raspberries)
- 1/2 cup heavy cream
- 1/4 cup granulated sweetener (e.g., Swerve or Erythritol)

Instructions:
1. In a blender, combine frozen berries, heavy cream, and sweetener. Blend until smooth.
2. Pour mixture into a bowl and serve immediately.

Note: You can also freeze the mixture in an ice cream maker or a shallow metal pan for a creamier texture.

Macro breakdown per serving (1/2 cup):

- Calories: 250
- Protein: 4g
- Fat: 22g
- Carbohydrates: 5g
- Fiber: 2g
- Net Carbs: 3g

Enjoy your delicious and easy 3-ingredient keto ice cream!

Global Cuisine

1. Korean Bibimbap

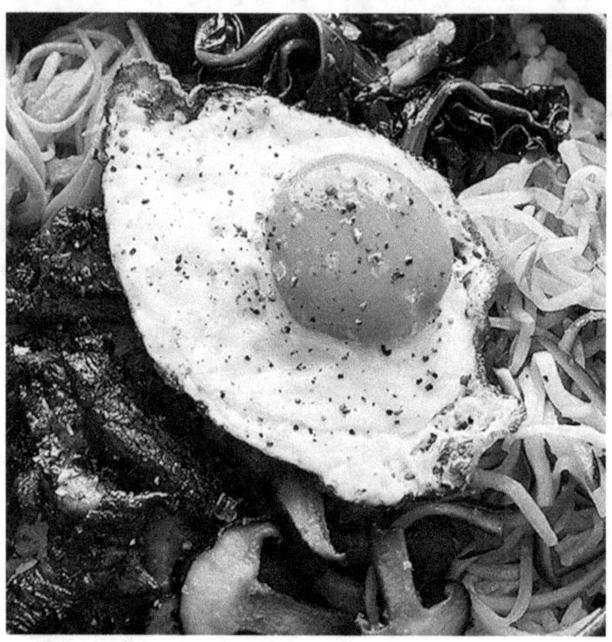

Ingredients:
- 1 cup cauliflower rice
- 1 cup mixed vegetables (bean sprouts, zucchini, carrots, mushrooms)
- 1/2 cup cooked beef (Bulgogi beef or ribeye)
- 1/4 cup fried egg
- 1/4 cup chopped green onions
- 1/4 cup diced cucumber
- 1/4 cup diced bell peppers
- 2 tbsp Gochujang sauce (Korean chili paste)

- 1 tsp soy sauce
- 1 tsp sesame oil
- Salt and pepper to taste

Instructions:
1. Cook the cauliflower rice and set aside.
2. In a separate pan, cook the mixed vegetables and beef.
3. In a small bowl, whisk together Gochujang sauce, soy sauce, and sesame oil.
4. In a large bowl, combine cooked cauliflower rice, vegetables, beef, and fried egg.
5. Drizzle the Gochujang sauce mixture over the top and garnish with green onions, cucumber, and bell peppers.

Macro breakdown (approximate):

- Calories: 350
- Protein: 25g
- Fat: 20g
- Carbohydrates: 5g
- Fiber: 5g
- Net Carbs: 0g

2. Indian Butter Chicken

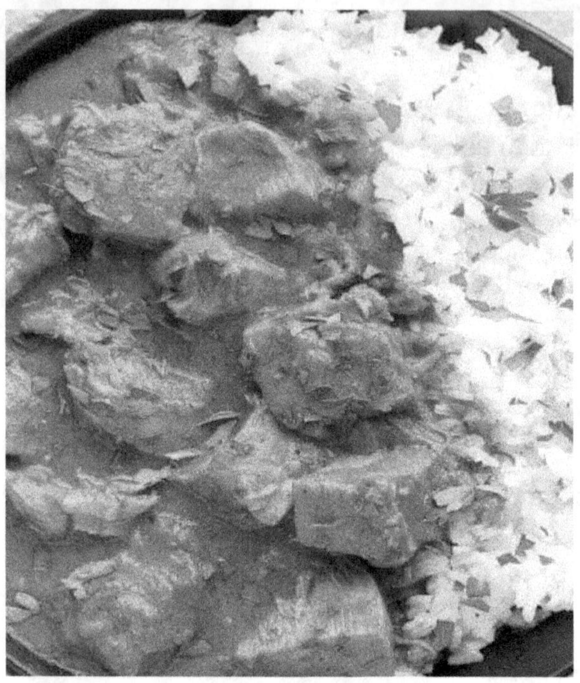

Ingredients:
- 1 1/2 pounds boneless, skinless chicken breast or thighs
- 1/2 cup plain Greek yogurt
- 2 tablespoons lemon juice
- 1 teaspoon garam masala
- 1/2 teaspoon ground cumin
- 1/2 teaspoon ground coriander
- 1/4 teaspoon ground cayenne pepper (optional)
- 1/4 cup butter
- 2 cloves garlic, minced
- 1 can (14 oz) diced tomatoes

- 1 cup chicken broth
- Salt and pepper, to taste
- Fresh cilantro, for garnish

Instructions:
1. In a large bowl, whisk together yogurt, lemon juice, garam masala, cumin, coriander, and cayenne pepper (if using).
2. Add the chicken and marinate for at least 30 minutes, or up to 2 hours in the refrigerator.
3. In a large skillet, melt 2 tablespoons of butter over medium heat. Remove the chicken from the marinade, letting any excess liquid drip off.
4. Cook the chicken until browned on all sides and cooked through, about 6-8 minutes.
5. Add the garlic, diced tomatoes, and chicken broth to the skillet. Stir to combine.
6. Reduce heat to low and simmer, uncovered, for 10-15 minutes or until the sauce has thickened slightly.
7. Stir in the remaining 2 tablespoons of butter until melted. Season with salt and pepper to taste.
8. Garnish with fresh cilantro and serve over cauliflower rice or vegetables.

Macro breakdown (approximate):

- Calories: 350
- Protein: 30g
- Fat: 25g
- Carbohydrates: 5g
- Fiber: 2g

- Net Carbs: 3g

3. Japanese Teriyaki Salmon

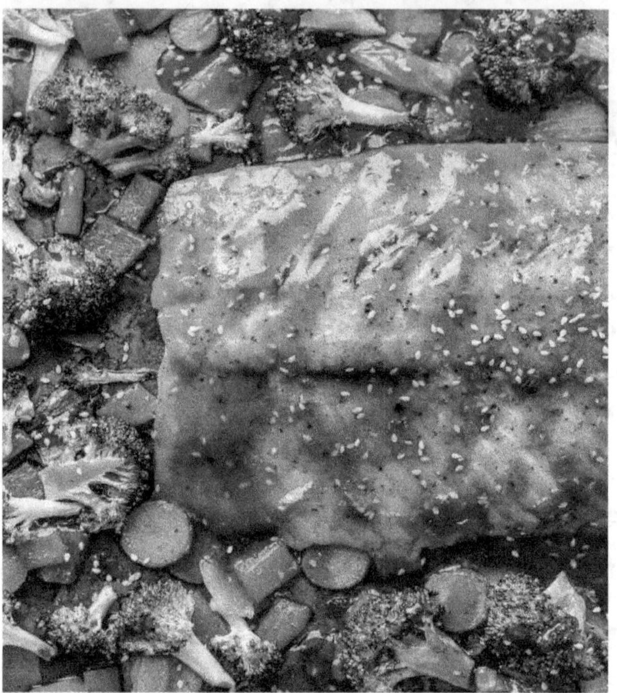

Ingredients:
- 4 salmon filets (6 oz each)
- 1/2 cup teriyaki sauce (make sure it's sugar-free)
- 1/4 cup avocado oil
- 2 cloves garlic, minced
- 1 tsp grated ginger
- 1 cup mixed vegetables (bell peppers, carrots, broccoli)
- Salt and pepper to taste

Instructions:
1. Preheat the oven to 400°F (200°C).
2. In a small bowl, whisk together teriyaki sauce, avocado oil, garlic, and ginger.
3. Place the salmon filets in a baking dish and brush the teriyaki mixture evenly over both sides.
4. Bake for 12-15 minutes or until cooked through.
5. Serve with roasted mixed vegetables.

Macro breakdown (approximate):

- Calories: 320
- Protein: 35g
- Fat: 20g
- Carbohydrates: 5g
- Fiber: 5g
- Net Carbs: 0g

4. Thai Green Curry

Ingredients:
- 2 cups mixed vegetables (bell peppers, Thai basil, bamboo shoots)
- 1 cup coconut milk
- 1/4 cup green curry paste
- 2 tbsp avocado oil
- 1 tsp grated ginger
- 1/2 cup cooked chicken or shrimp
- 1/4 cup chopped fresh cilantro
- Salt and pepper to taste
- 1/4 cup chopped macadamia nuts (optional)

Instructions:
1. In a large skillet, heat avocado oil over medium heat.
2. Add green curry paste and cook, stirring constantly, for 1 minute.
3. Add coconut milk, mixed vegetables, ginger, and protein (chicken or shrimp). Stir to combine.
4. Reduce heat to low and simmer, uncovered, for 10-15 minutes or until vegetables are tender.
5. Stir in chopped cilantro and macadamia nuts (if using). Season with salt and pepper to taste.
6. Serve hot over cauliflower rice or vegetables.

Macro breakdown (approximate):

- Calories: 350
- Protein: 25g
- Fat: 25g
- Carbohydrates: 5g
- Fiber: 5g
- Net Carbs: 0g

5. Vietnamese Pho

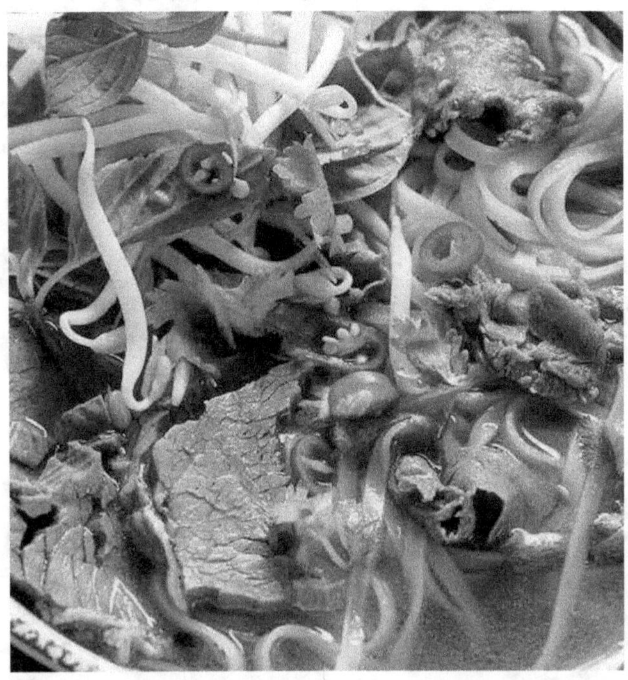

Ingredients:
- 1 pound beef (rare steak or brisket), sliced thinly
- 2 cups beef broth (make sure it's sugar-free)
- 1 cup zucchini noodles (or shirataki noodles)
- 1/4 cup chopped onion
- 1/4 cup chopped cilantro
- 1/4 cup sliced lime
- 2 cloves garlic, minced
- 1 tsp ground ginger
- Salt and pepper to taste
- Optional: 1/4 cup chopped bean sprouts, 1/4 cup
sliced mushrooms

Instructions:
1. In a large pot, combine beef broth, onion, cilantro, lime juice, garlic, and ginger. Bring to a boil, then reduce heat and simmer.
2. Cook the zucchini noodles according to package instructions. Drain and set aside.
3. Add the sliced beef to the pot and cook for 2-3 minutes, or until cooked to your liking.
4. Assemble the Pho by placing the zucchini noodles in a bowl, then adding the beef and hot broth. Garnish with bean sprouts and mushrooms (if using).

Macro breakdown (approximate):

- Calories: 300
- Protein: 30g
- Fat: 20g
- Carbohydrates: 5g
- Fiber: 5g
- Net Carbs: 0g

6. Chinese Beef And Broccoli

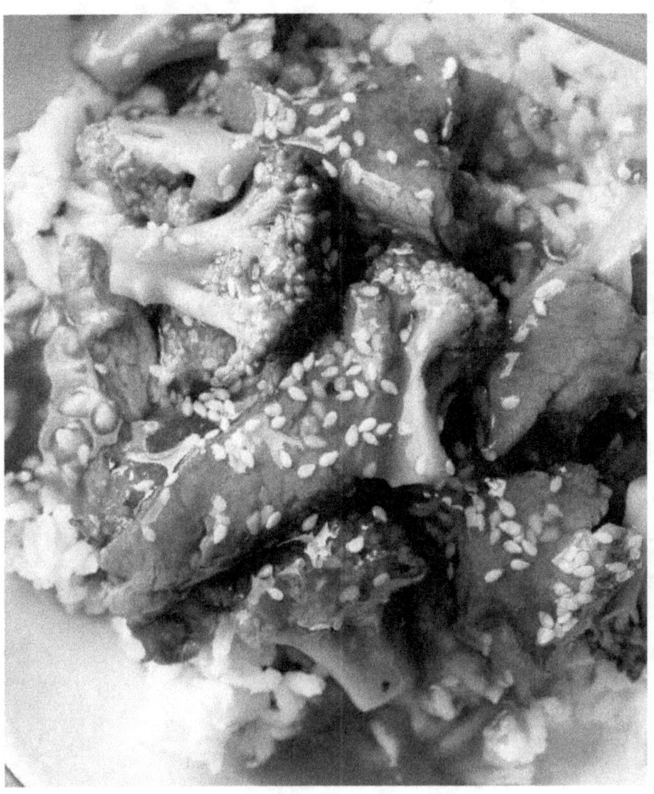

Ingredients:

- 1 pound beef (sirloin or ribeye), sliced
- 2 cups broccoli florets
- 1/4 cup coconut aminos (or low-carb soy sauce)
- 1/4 cup avocado oil
- 2 cloves garlic, minced
- 1 tsp grated ginger
- Salt and pepper to taste

Instructions:

1. In a large skillet, heat avocado oil over medium-high heat.
2. Add beef and cook until browned, about 3-4 minutes. Remove from the skillet.
3. Add broccoli, garlic, and ginger to the skillet. Cook until broccoli is tender, about 3-4 minutes.
4. In a small bowl, whisk together coconut aminos and 1 tablespoon water. Pour into the skillet and stir to combine.
5. Return beef to the skillet and cook for an additional 1-2 minutes.
6. Serve hot over cauliflower rice or vegetables.

Macro breakdown (approximate):

- Calories: 300
- Protein: 30g
- Fat: 20g
- Carbohydrates: 5g
- Fiber: 5g
- Net Carbs: 0g

7. Mexican Carnitas

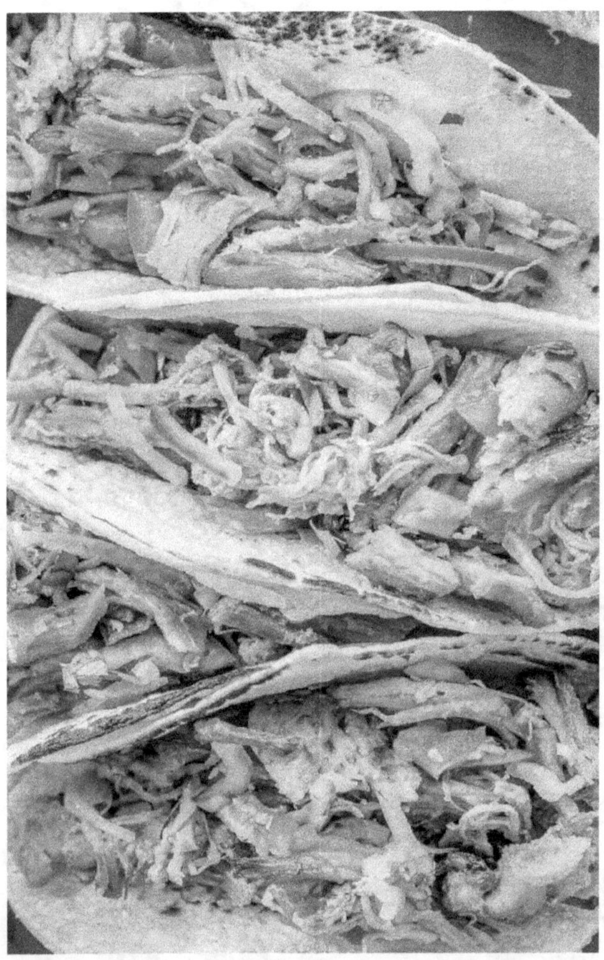

Ingredients:

- 2 pounds pork shoulder, cut into large chunks
- 1/4 cup lard or avocado oil
- 1/4 cup freshly squeezed orange juice
- 1/4 cup freshly squeezed lime juice

- 2 cloves garlic, minced
- 1 tsp dried oregano
- Salt and pepper to taste
- 1 cup mixed vegetables (bell peppers, onions, tomatoes)
- 4 low-carb tortillas (optional)

Instructions:

1. In a large Dutch oven, heat lard or avocado oil over medium heat.
2. Add pork chunks and cook until browned on all sides, about 5 minutes.
3. Add orange and lime juice, garlic, and oregano. Cover and simmer for 2-3 hours or until tender.
4. Shred the pork with two forks and stir in mixed vegetables.
5. Serve with low-carb tortillas (if using) and your favorite toppings like avocado, sour cream, and salsa.

Macro breakdown (approximate):

- Calories: 350
- Protein: 30g
- Fat: 25g
- Carbohydrates: 5g
- Fiber: 5g
- Net Carbs: 0g

8. Greek Gyro

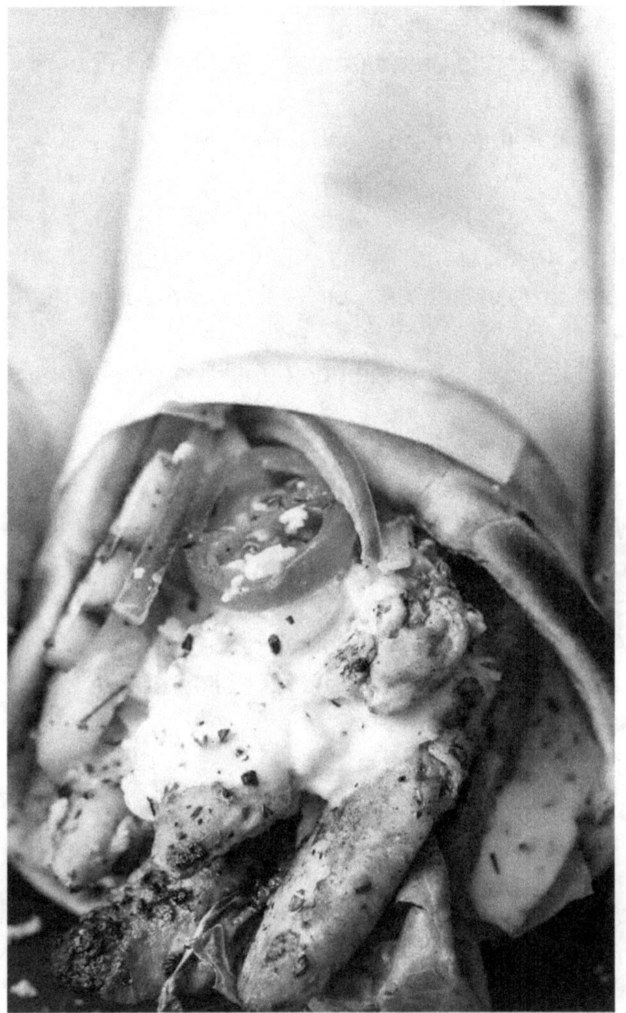

Ingredients:
- 1 pound lamb or beef, sliced thinly
- 1/4 cup olive oil
- 2 cloves garlic, minced

- 1 tsp dried oregano
- 1 tsp lemon zest
- Salt and pepper to taste
- 4 low-carb pita bread (made with almond flour or coconut flour)
- Tzatziki sauce (made with Greek yogurt, cucumber, garlic, and dill)

Instructions:

1. In a large skillet, heat olive oil over medium-high heat.
2. Add lamb or beef and cook until browned, about 3-4 minutes.
3. Add garlic, oregano, and lemon zest. Cook for an additional minute.
4. Warm the low-carb pita bread by wrapping it in a damp paper towel and microwaving for 20-30 seconds.
5. Assemble the Gyro by placing the meat mixture on the pita bread, followed by a dollop of Tzatziki sauce and your choice of toppings (e.g., tomato, onion, cucumber, feta cheese).

Macro breakdown (approximate):

- Calories: 350
- Protein: 30g
- Fat: 25g
- Carbohydrates: 5g
- Fiber: 5g
- Net Carbs: 0g

9. Vietnamese Ceviche

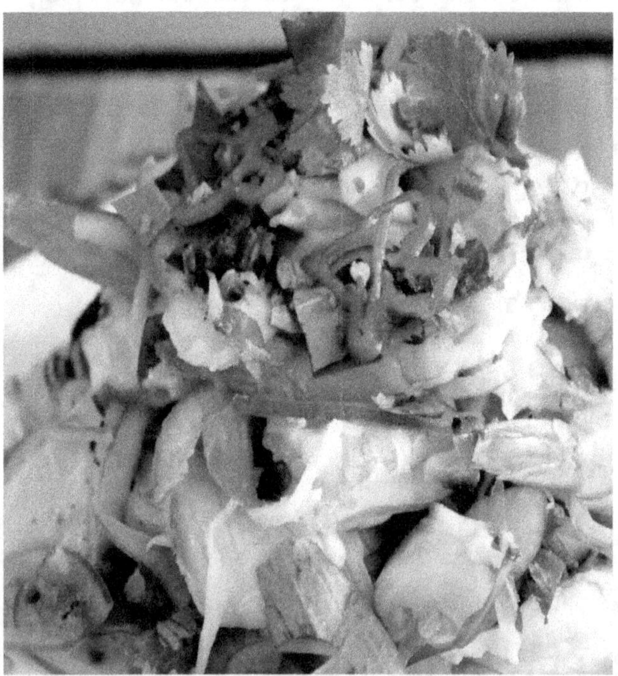

Ingredients:
- 1 pound fish (halibut or snapper), sliced into thin pieces
- 1/2 cup freshly squeezed lime juice
- 1/4 cup fish sauce (make sure it's sugar-free)
- 1/4 cup chopped cilantro
- 1/4 cup chopped mint leaves
- 1/4 cup sliced red onion
- 1/4 cup sliced bell peppers
- 2 cloves garlic, minced
- Salt and pepper to taste

Instructions:

1. In a large bowl, combine fish slices, lime juice, fish sauce, cilantro, mint leaves, red onion, bell peppers, and garlic.
2. Refrigerate for at least 30 minutes to allow the fish to "cook" in the lime juice.
3. Serve chilled, garnished with additional cilantro and mint leaves if desired.

Macro breakdown (approximate):

- Calories: 250
- Protein: 30g
- Fat: 15g
- Carbohydrates: 5g
- Fiber: 5g
- Net Carbs: 0g

10. Peruvian Ceviche

Ingredients:
- 1 pound fresh seafood (halibut, shrimp, scallops)
- 1/2 cup freshly squeezed lime juice
- 1/4 cup chopped red onion
- 1/4 cup chopped fresh cilantro
- 1/4 cup chopped fresh tomatoes
- 1 aji amarillo pepper, seeded and chopped
- Salt and pepper to taste

Instructions:

1. Cut the seafood into small pieces and place in a large bowl.

2. Pour lime juice over the seafood and refrigerate
for at least 30 minutes to marinate.
3. Add chopped onion, cilantro, tomatoes, and aji
amarillo pepper to the bowl.
4. Stir to combine and season with salt and pepper
to taste.
5. Serve immediately, garnished with additional
cilantro if desired.

Macro breakdown (approximate):

- Calories: 200
- Protein: 30g
- Fat: 10g
- Carbohydrates: 5g
- Fiber: 5g
- Net Carbs: 0g

Drinks

1. Strawberry Keto Smoothie

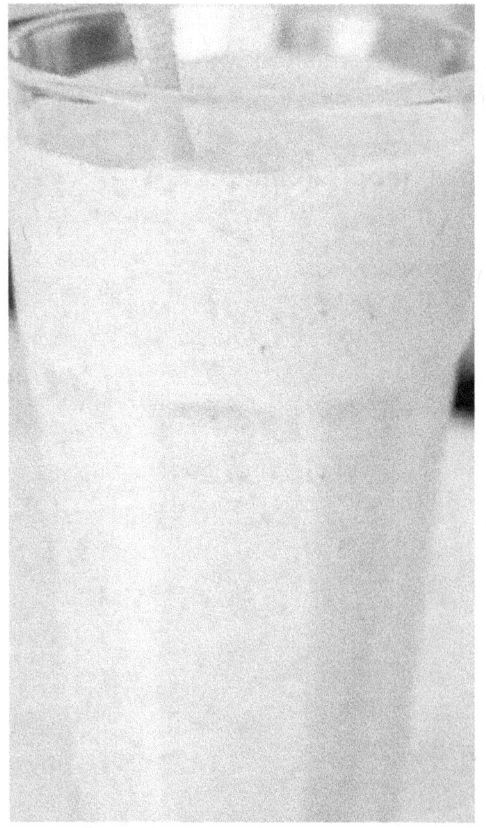

Ingredients:
- 1/2 cup frozen strawberries
- 1/2 cup unsweetened almond milk
- 1/4 cup heavy cream
- 1 scoop vanilla protein powder

- 1/2 teaspoon sweetener (like stevia or erythritol)
- Ice cubes (as needed)

Instructions:
1. Add all ingredients to a blender and blend until smooth.
2. Taste and adjust sweetness as needed.
3. Pour into a glass and serve immediately.

Macro breakdown (approximate):

- Calories: 350
- Protein: 25g
- Fat: 25g
- Carbohydrates: 5g
- Fiber: 2g
- Net Carbs: 3g

2. Mocha Protein Shake

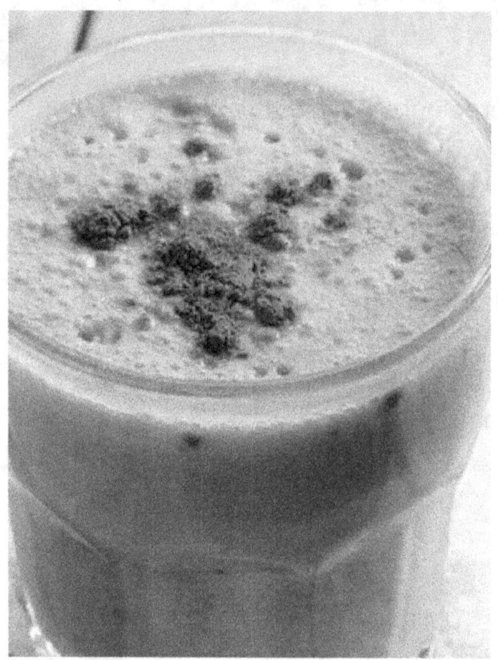

Ingredients:
- 1 scoop chocolate protein powder
- 1/2 cup unsweetened almond milk
- 1/4 cup heavy cream
- 1/2 teaspoon instant coffee powder
- 1/2 teaspoon sweetener (like stevia or erythritol)
- Ice cubes (as needed)

Instructions:
1. Add all ingredients to a blender and blend until smooth.
2. Taste and adjust sweetness as needed.
3. Pour into a glass and serve immediately.

Macro breakdown (approximate):

- Calories: 300
- Protein: 20g
- Fat: 20g
- Carbohydrates: 5g
- Fiber: 2g
- Net Carbs: 3g

You can also add other ingredients to customize your shake, such as:

- A handful of ice to thicken the shake
- A sprinkle of cinnamon or cocoa powder for extra flavor
- A shot of espresso for an extra caffeine boost

3. Blueberry Lemonade Smoothie

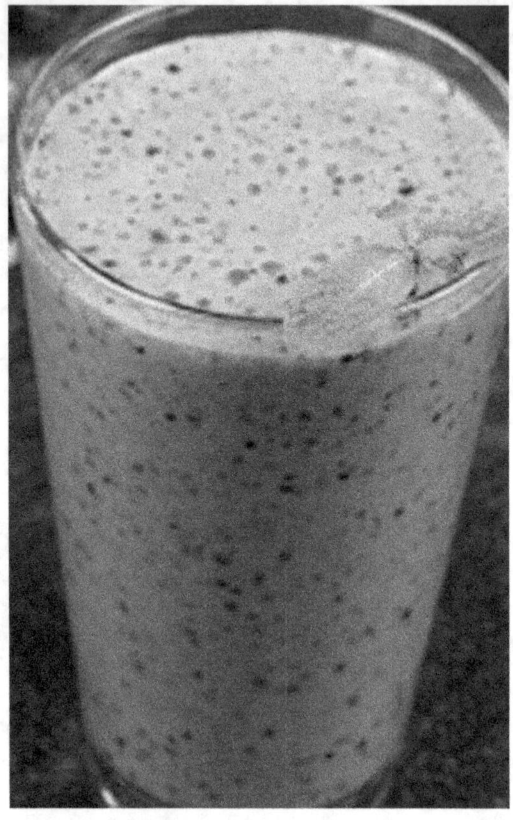

Ingredients:
- 1/2 cup frozen blueberries
- 1/2 cup unsweetened almond milk
- 1/4 cup freshly squeezed lemon juice
- 1 scoop vanilla protein powder
- 1/2 teaspoon sweetener (like stevia or erythritol)
- Ice cubes (as needed)

Instructions:

1. Add all ingredients to a blender and blend until smooth.
2. Taste and adjust sweetness as needed.
3. Pour into a glass and serve immediately.

Macro breakdown (approximate):

- Calories: 250
- Protein: 20g
- Fat: 15g
- Carbohydrates: 5g
- Fiber: 2g
- Net Carbs: 3g

You can also add other ingredients to customize your smoothie, such as:

- A handful of spinach or kale for a green smoothie
- A slice of fresh pineapple or mango for extra flavor
- A sprinkle of lemon zest for extra citrus flavor

4. Peanut Butter Banana Shake

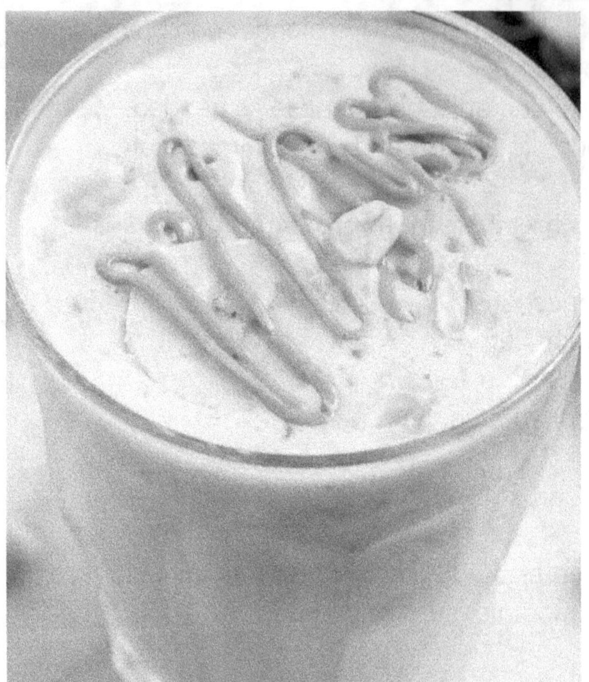

Ingredients:

- 1 scoop vanilla protein powder
- 1/2 banana
- 2 tablespoons natural peanut butter
- 1/2 cup unsweetened almond milk
- 1/2 teaspoon sweetener (like stevia or erythritol)
- Ice cubes (as needed)

Instructions:

1. Add all ingredients to a blender and blend until smooth.
2. Taste and adjust sweetness as needed.

3. Pour into a glass and serve immediately.

Macro breakdown (approximate):

- Calories: 350
- Protein: 20g
- Fat: 25g
- Carbohydrates: 5g
- Fiber: 2g
- Net Carbs: 3g

You can also add other ingredients to customize your shake, such as:

- A handful of ice to thicken the shake
- A sprinkle of cinnamon or nutmeg for extra flavor
- A shot of espresso for an extra caffeine boost

5. Pina Colada Protein Smoothie

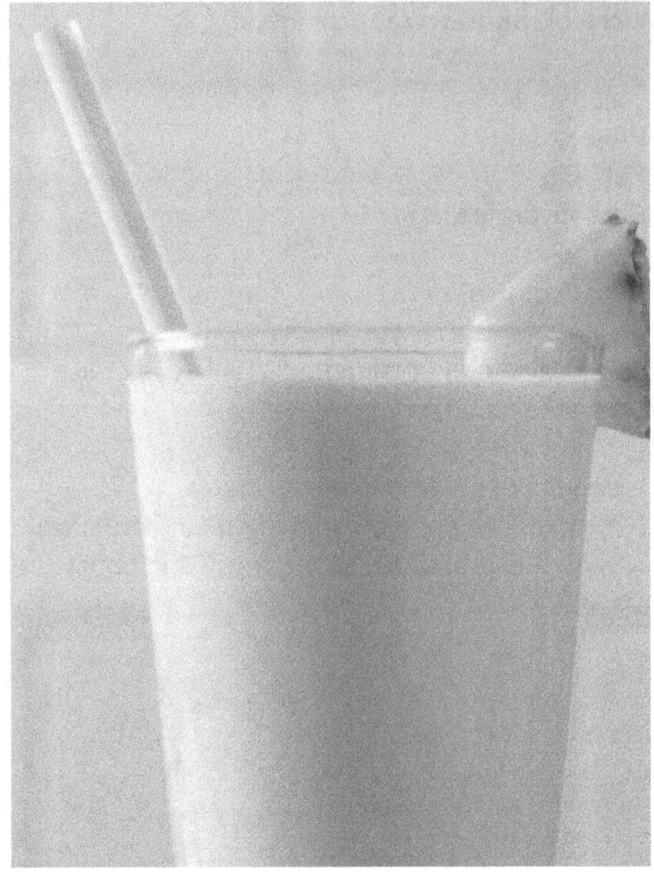

Ingredients:
- 1 scoop vanilla protein powder
- 1/2 cup frozen pineapple
- 1/4 cup unsweetened coconut milk
- 1/4 cup unsweetened almond milk
- 1/2 teaspoon sweetener (like stevia or erythritol)
- Ice cubes (as needed)

Instructions:
1. Add all ingredients to a blender and blend until smooth.
2. Taste and adjust sweetness as needed.
3. Pour into a glass and serve immediately.

Macro breakdown (approximate):

- Calories: 300
- Protein: 20g
- Fat: 20g
- Carbohydrates: 5g
- Fiber: 2g
- Net Carbs: 3g

You can also add other ingredients to customize your smoothie, such as:

- A sprinkle of shredded coconut for extra texture
- A slice of fresh mango for extra flavor
- A handful of spinach or kale for a green smoothie

6. Vodka Soda

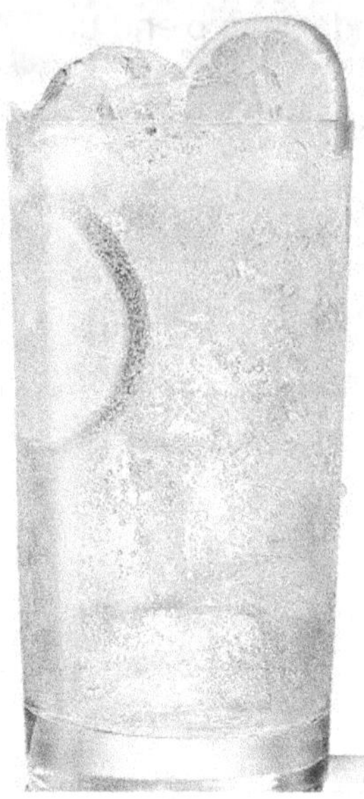

Ingredients:
- 1.5 oz vodka
- 4 oz soda water
- Lime wedge (optional)

Instructions:
1. Fill a highball glass with ice.
2. Pour in the vodka.
3. Top with soda water.
4. Squeeze in a lime wedge, if desired.
5. Stir briefly.
6. Serve and enjoy!

Macro breakdown (approximate):

- Calories: 96
- Protein: 0g
- Fat: 0g
- Carbohydrates: 0g
- Fiber: 0g
- Net Carbs: 0g

The Vodka Soda is a classic, low-carb cocktail that's easy to make and refreshing to drink. The soda water adds a bit of fizz without adding any carbs.

7. Virgin Mojito

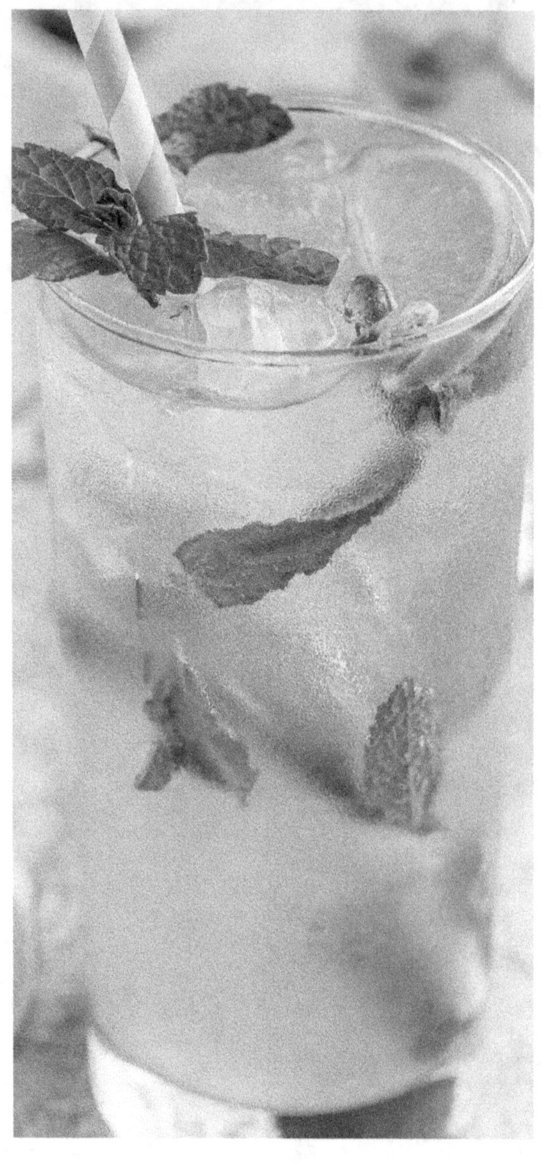

Ingredients:
- 1 sprig of fresh mint leaves
- 1 lime, juiced
- 4 oz soda water
- Ice cubes

Instructions:
1. In a tall glass, gently press the mint leaves with a muddler or the back of a spoon to release the oils and flavor.
2. Add the lime juice and stir to combine.
3. Fill the glass with ice cubes.
4. Top with soda water and stir briefly.
5. Garnish with a sprig of fresh mint and serve.

Macro breakdown (approximate):

- Calories: 0
- Protein: 0g
- Fat: 0g
- Carbohydrates: 0g
- Fiber: 0g
- Net Carbs: 0g

The Virgin Mojito is a refreshing, low-carb mocktail that's perfect for warm weather or any time you want a light, crisp drink. The mint and lime flavors are a great combination!

8. Gin & Tonic

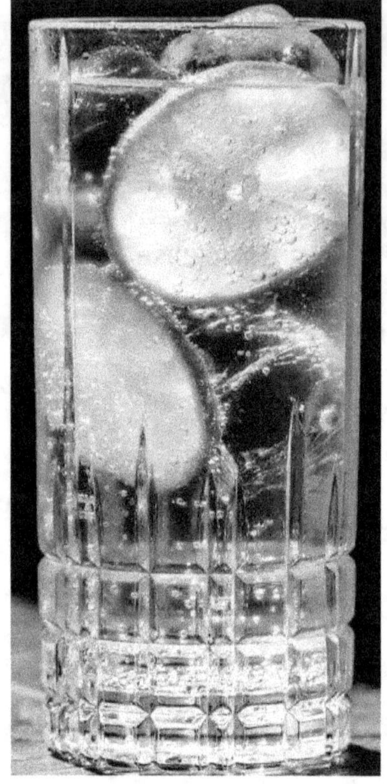

Ingredients:

- 1.5 oz gin
- 4 oz tonic water
- Lime wedge (optional)

Instructions:

1. Fill a highball glass with ice.
2. Pour in the gin.
3. Top with tonic water.
4. Squeeze in a lime wedge, if desired.

5. Stir briefly.
6. Serve and enjoy!

Macro breakdown (approximate):

- Calories: 120
- Protein: 0g
- Fat: 0g
- Carbohydrates: 5g
- Fiber: 0g
- Net Carbs: 5g

The Gin & Tonic is a classic cocktail that's easy to make and refreshing to drink. The tonic water adds a bit of sweetness and bitterness to balance out the gin.
Note: Some tonic waters may contain more carbs than others, so be sure to check the label if you're tracking your carb intake.

9. Cucumber Lime Refresher

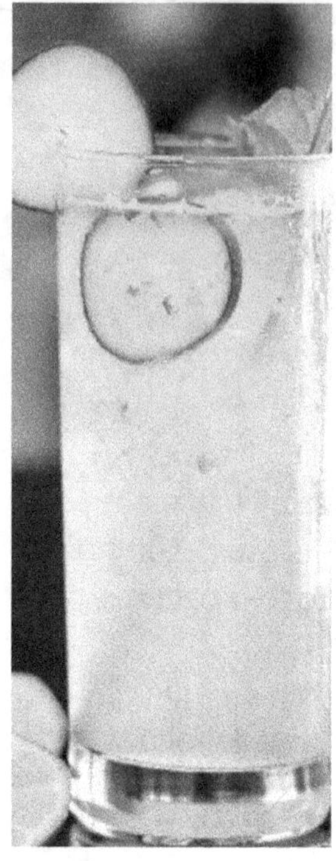

Ingredients:
- 1/2 cucumber, sliced
- 1 lime, juiced
- 4 oz soda water
- Ice cubes

Instructions:
1. In a tall glass, add the cucumber slices and lime juice.
2. Fill the glass with ice cubes.
3. Top with soda water and stir briefly.

4. Garnish with a cucumber slice or lime wedge, if
desired.
5. Serve and enjoy!

Macro breakdown (approximate):

- Calories: 16
- Protein: 0g
- Fat: 0g
- Carbohydrates: 4g
- Fiber: 1g
- Net Carbs: 3g

The Cucumber Lime Refresher is a light, refreshing
mocktail that's perfect for hot summer days or any
time you want a low-calorie, low-carb drink. The
cucumber adds a cool, refreshing flavor that pairs
well with the lime juice.

10. Low-Carb Margarita

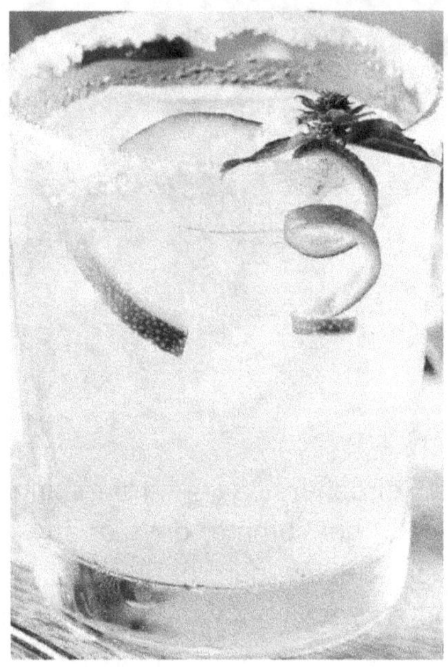

Ingredients:
- 2 oz tequila
- 1 oz fresh lime juice
- 1/2 oz triple sec (or low-carb orange liqueur)
- Salt rim (optional)

Instructions:
1. Rim a rocks glass with salt, if desired.
2. Fill a cocktail shaker with ice.
3. Add the tequila, lime juice, and triple sec.
4. Shake until chilled.
5. Strain into the prepared glass.
6. Garnish with a lime wedge, if desired.

Macro breakdown (approximate):

- Calories: 160
- Protein: 0g
- Fat: 0g
- Carbohydrates: 5g
- Fiber: 0g
- Net Carbs: 5g

The Low-Carb Margarita is a tangy and refreshing twist on the classic cocktail. By using a low-carb orange liqueur, you can enjoy the flavor without the added sugar. **Note:** Some triple sec brands may contain more carbs than others, so be sure to check the label if you're tracking your carb intake.

Chapter Five

Meal Planning Tips

1. Set your goals: Define your dietary needs and preferences (e.g., vegetarian, gluten-free, low-carb).

2. Plan around sales: Check weekly grocery ads and plan meals around sale items.

3. Shop your pantry first: Use ingredients you already have to reduce waste and save money.

4. Keep it simple: Choose simple recipes with fewer ingredients.

5. Cook in bulk: Prepare large batches of rice, beans, or grains for future meals.

6. Make a grocery list: Write down the ingredients you need and stick to your list.

7. Be flexible: Swap out ingredients or interchange recipes if needed.

8. Consider one-pot meals: Choose recipes that cook in one pot for easy cleanup.

9. Leftovers are your friend: Use leftovers to reduce food waste and save time.

10. Review and adjust: Regularly review your meal plan and make adjustments as needed.

Remember, meal planning is a process, and it may take some time to figure out what works best for you. Be patient, stay consistent and be happy cooking!

Grocery Shopping Tips And Tricks

1. Make a list and stick to it: Avoid impulse buys and stay focused on what you need.

2. Plan meals around sales: Check weekly ads and plan meals around discounted items.

3. Shop the perimeter of the store: Fresh produce, meats, and dairy products are often located on the perimeter.

4. Buy in bulk: Purchase non-perishable items in bulk to save money and reduce waste.

5. Use coupons and discount codes: Take advantage of digital coupons, discount codes, and cashback apps.

6. Shop at local markets or farmers' markets: Support local farmers and find fresh, unique ingredients.

7. Avoid shopping when you're hungry: Eat before shopping to avoid impulse buys and stick to your list.

8. Use unit prices: Compare prices between brands and sizes by checking the unit price (price per ounce or pound).

9. Don't shop at high-end stores: Consider shopping at discount stores or dollar stores for non-perishable items.

10. Buy in season: Purchase produce in season to save money and ensure freshness.

11. Use store loyalty programs: Sign up for loyalty programs to earn rewards, discounts, and exclusive offers.

Remember, grocery shopping is a skill that takes practice, so don't be too hard on yourself if you don't get it right immediately. Happy shopping!

Conclusion

As we come to the end of this culinary journey, we hope that the recipes and tips provided in this book have inspired you to embrace a low-carb lifestyle and experience the numerous health benefits that come with it.

Throughout this book, we've shown you that low-carb cooking doesn't have to be boring or restrictive. With a little creativity and experimentation, you can create delicious and satisfying meals that are both healthy and flavorful. From breakfast to dinner, and from snacks to desserts, we've covered it all.

By following the recipes in this book, you've learned how to make delicious low-carb versions of your favorite comfort foods, incorporate healthy fats and proteins into your meals, use vegetables and fruits in creative and tasty ways, and even make low-carb baking and desserts a reality. You've also gained valuable tips and tricks for success on a low-carb diet, from stocking your pantry and fridge with low-carb essentials to planning and preparing meals for the week.

We've also shared stories of people who have transformed their lives with a low-carb lifestyle, and we hope that their stories have inspired and motivated you to continue on your own journey. Whether you're looking to improve your health, increase your energy levels, or simply feel better in your own skin, we believe that a low-carb lifestyle can help you achieve your goals.

Of course, we know that it's not always easy. There will be challenges and setbacks along the way, and there will be times when you feel like giving up. But we encourage you to stay the course, to keep pushing forward even when it gets tough. Because the truth is, the benefits of a low-carb lifestyle far outweigh the costs. And with the recipes and tips in this book, you have everything you need to succeed.

So what's next? We encourage you to keep exploring the world of low-carb cooking, to try new recipes and ingredients, and to experiment with different flavors and techniques. Don't be afraid to try new things and to make mistakes – that's where the magic happens!

We also encourage you to share your own low-carb journey with others, to inspire and motivate them to make positive changes in their own lives. Whether it's through social media, a blog, or simply sharing your story with friends and family, we believe that your journey can make a difference in the lives of others.

In conclusion, we hope that this book has been a valuable resource on your journey to a healthier, happier you. We hope that the recipes and tips we've shared have inspired you to take control of your health and to make positive changes in your life. And we hope that you'll continue to join us on this journey, as we explore the many benefits of a low-carb lifestyle. Happy cooking and happy health

Tips For Success On A Low-Carb Diet

1. Set clear goals: Define your goals and why you want to follow a low-carb diet. This will help you stay motivated and focused.

2. Plan ahead: Meal prep, grocery shop, and plan your meals for the week to avoid last-minute high-carb choices.

3. Focus on whole foods: Emphasize whole, unprocessed foods like meats, fish, eggs, veggies, nuts, and seeds.

4. Read labels: Be aware of hidden carbs in packaged foods and read labels carefully.

5. Stay hydrated: Drink plenty of water and consider increasing your salt intake to help your body adapt.

6. Be mindful of portion sizes: Even low-carb foods can lead to weight gain if consumed in excess.

7. Don't be too hard on yourself: Allow for occasional slip-ups and get back on track without guilt.

8. Get support: Join a low-carb community or find a support buddy for motivation and encouragement.

9. Monitor progress: Track your progress through measurements, weight, and blood work to stay motivated.

10. Be patient: Adaptation to a low-carb diet can take time, so be patient and don't get discouraged by initial side effects.

11. Get enough sleep: Poor sleep can disrupt hormones and metabolism, making it harder to succeed on a low-carb diet.

12. Stay positive: Focus on the benefits and enjoy the journey to a healthier, happier you!

Remember, everyone is unique, and it may take some trial and error to find what works best for you. Stay committed, and don't hesitate to seek guidance from a healthcare professional if needed. Good luck

Appendix

7-Days Meal Plan

Day 1:
- Breakfast: Scrambled eggs with spinach and avocado
- Lunch: Grilled chicken breast with roasted vegetables
- Dinner: Baked salmon with cauliflower rice and green beans

Day 2:
- Breakfast: Low-carb protein smoothie with almond milk and berries
- Lunch: Turkey lettuce wraps with avocado and tomato
- Dinner: Grilled steak with roasted Brussels sprouts and sweet potato

Day 3:
- Breakfast: Low-carb pancakes made with almond flour and topped with butter and sugar-free syrup
- Lunch: Chicken Caesar salad with romaine lettuce and parmesan cheese
- Dinner: Pork chops with roasted broccoli and a side salad

Day 4:
- Breakfast: Spinach and feta omelet

- Lunch: Grilled chicken breast with mixed greens
and a vinaigrette dressing
- Dinner: Beef stir-fry with vegetables and
cauliflower rice

Day 5:
- Breakfast: Low-carb yogurt with berries and
chopped nuts
- Lunch: Chicken salad with celery and tomato
- Dinner: Grilled chicken breast with roasted
asparagus and a side salad

Day 6:
- Breakfast: Breakfast burrito with scrambled eggs,
avocado, and tomato
- Lunch: Turkey and cheese roll-ups with lettuce
and tomato
- Dinner: Baked chicken thighs with roasted bell
peppers and a side salad

Day 7:
- Breakfast: Low-carb waffles made with almond
flour and topped with butter and sugar-free syrup
- Lunch: Grilled chicken Caesar salad
- Dinner: Pork tenderloin with roasted Brussels
sprouts and sweet potato

Grocery Shopping List And Pantry Staples

Meat and Poultry:

- Grass-fed beef
- Pasture-raised chicken
- Wild-caught fish
- Pork
- Lamb
- Turkey
- Bacon
- Sausages

Vegetables:
- Leafy greens (spinach, kale, lettuce)
- Broccoli
- Cauliflower
- Avocado
- Bell peppers
- Cucumbers
- Tomatoes
- Mushrooms
- Asparagus
- Zucchini

Low-Carb Fruits:
- Berries (strawberries, blueberries, raspberries)
- Citrus fruits (oranges, lemons, limes)
- Avocado (yes, it's a fruit!)
- Tomatoes (technically a fruit, but often thought of as a veggie)

Dairy and Eggs:
- Full-fat cheese (cheddar, parmesan, feta)
- Greek yogurt
- Cottage cheese

- Eggs
- Heavy cream

Nuts and Seeds:
- Almonds
- Walnuts
- Chia seeds
- Flax seeds
- Pumpkin seeds
- Coconut flakes

Pantry Staples:
- Almond flour
- Coconut flour
- Olive oil
- Avocado oil
- Salt
- Pepper
- Garlic powder
- Onion powder
- Paprika
- Cumin
- Coriander
- Turmeric
- Ginger
- Bone broth
- Canned tomatoes
- Canned tuna
- Canned salmon

Low-Carb Grains:
- Almond flour tortillas

- Coconut flour bread
- Cauliflower rice
- Zucchini noodles
- Shirataki noodles

Condiments:
- Sugar-free ketchup
- Sugar-free mayonnaise
- Mustard
- Hot sauce
- Salsa
- Guacamole

Conversion Chart

Volume Conversions:
- 1 cup (cups) = 8 fluid ounces (fl oz) = 237 milliliters (mL)
- 1/2 cup = 4 fl oz = 118 mL
- 1/3 cup = 3 fl oz = 79 mL
- 1/4 cup = 2 fl oz = 59 mL

Weight Conversions:
- 1 pound (lb) = 16 ounces (oz) = 450 grams (g)
- 1/2 lb = 8 oz = 225 g
- 1/3 lb = 5.3 oz = 150 g
- 1/4 lb = 4 oz = 115 g

Length Conversions:

- 1 inch (in) = 2.54 centimeters (cm)

Cooking Conversions:
- 1 tablespoon (tbsp) = 3 teaspoons (tsp)
- 1 teaspoon = 5 milliliters (mL)

Low-Carb Conversions:
- 1 cup sugar = 1/2 cup sugar substitute (e.g. Swerve, Erythritol)
- 1 cup all-purpose flour = 1/2 cup almond flour or coconut flour

Meal Planning Templates

- Monday
  - Breakfast:

____

____

____

____

  - Lunch:

____

____

____

____

  -

Dinner:_________________________________

____

____

____

  - Snack:

____

____

____ 271

____

- Tuesday

-

Breakfast:____

____

____

____

- Lunch:

____

____

____

____

-

Dinner:____

____

____

____

- Snack:

____

____

____

____

- Wednesday

-

Breakfast:____

____

____

____

- Lunch:

____

____

____

____

-

Dinner:________________________________

____

____

____

- Snack:

____

____

____

____

- Thursday
  - Breakfast:

____

____

____

____

  - Lunch:

____

____

____

____

-

Dinner:________________________________

____

____

____

- Snack:

____

____

____

____

- Friday
-
Breakfast:_______________________________

____

____

____

- Lunch:

____

____

____

____
-
Dinner:_______________________________

____

____

____

- Snack:

____

____

____

____

- Saturday
-
Breakfast:_______________________________

____

- Lunch:

- Dinner:

- Snack:

- **Sunday**
  - Breakfast:

- Lunch:

- Dinner:

- Snack: